T0259344

Hepatitis B Virus

Editors

TARIK ASSELAH
PATRICK MARCELLIN

CLINICS IN LIVER DISEASE

www.liver.theclinics.com

Consulting Editor
NORMAN GITLIN

August 2013 • Volume 17 • Number 3

ELSEVIER

1600 John F. Kennedy Boulevard • Suite 1800 • Philadelphia, Pennsylvania, 19103-2899

http://www.theclinics.com

CLINICS IN LIVER DISEASE Volume 17, Number 3
August 2013 ISSN 1089-3261, ISBN-13: 978-0-323-18608-7

Editor: Kerry Holland

Clinics in Liver Disease (ISSN 1089-3261) is published quarterly by Elsevier Inc., 360 Park Avenue South, New York, NY 10010-1710. Months of issue are February, May, August, and November. Business and Editorial Offices: 1600 John F. Kennedy Blvd., Ste. 1800, Philadelphia, PA 19103-2899. Customer Service Office: 3251 Riverport Lane, Maryland Heights, MO 63043. Periodicals postage paid at New York, NY and additional mailing offices. Subscription prices are $282.00 per year (U.S. individuals), $139.00 per year (U.S. student/resident), $387.00 per year (U.S. institutions), $374.00 per year (foreign individuals), $192.00 per year (foreign student/resident), $465.00 per year (foreign instituitions), $326.00 per year (Canadian individuals), $192.00 per year (Canadian student/resident), and $465.00 per year (Canadian institutions). Foreign air speed delivery is included in all *Clinics* subscription prices. All prices are subject to change without notice. **POSTMASTER:** Send address changes to *Clinics in Liver Disease*, Elsevier Health Sciences Division, Subscription Customer Service, 3251 Riverport Lane, Maryland Heights, MO 63043. **Customer Service: Telephone: 1-800-654-2452 (U.S. and Canada); 314-447-8871 (outside U.S. and Canada). Fax: 314-447-8029. E-mail: journalscustomer service-usa@elsevier.com (for print support); journalsonlinesupport-usa@elsevier.com (for online support).**

Reprints. For copies of 100 or more of articles in this publication, please contact the Commercial Reprints Department, Elsevier Inc., 360 Park Avenue South, New York, NY 10010-1710. Tel.: 212-633-3812; Fax: 212-462-1935; E-mail: reprints@elsevier.com.

Clinics in Liver Disease is covered in *MEDLINE/PubMed (Index Medicus)*, Science Citation Index Expanded, Journal Citation Reports/Science Edition, and Current Contents/Clinical Medicine.

Printed and bound by CPI Group (UK) Ltd, Croydon, CR0 4YY
Transferred to digital print 2013

Contributors

CONSULTING EDITOR

NORMAN GITLIN, MD, FRCP (LONDON), FRCPE (EDINBURGH), FACG, FACP
Formerly, Professor of Medicine, Chief of Hepatology, Emory University; Currently, Consultant, Atlanta Gastroenterology Associates, Atlanta, Georgia

EDITORS

TARIK ASSELAH, MD, PhD
Professor of Medicine, University Paris Diderot, Department of Hepatology, Hôpital Beaujon, Clichy, France

PATRICK MARCELLIN, MD, PhD
Professor of Medicine, University Paris Diderot, Department of Hepatology, Hôpital Beaujon, Clichy, France

AUTHORS

SEYED MOAYED ALAVIAN, MD
Middle East Liver Diseases Center (MELD Center), Teheran, Iran

TARIK ASSELAH, MD, PhD
Professor of Medicine, University Paris Diderot, Department of Hepatology, Hôpital Beaujon, Clichy, France

PABLO BARREIRO, MD, PhD
Department of Infectious Diseases, Hospital Carlos III, Madrid, Spain

MASSIMO COLOMBO, MD
1st Division of Gastroenterology, A.M. and A. Migliavacca Center for Liver Disease, Fondazione IRCCS Ca' Granda Maggiore Hospital, Università degli Studi di Milano, Milan, Italy

MASSIMO IAVARONE, MD
1st Division of Gastroenterology, A.M. and A. Migliavacca Center for Liver Disease, Fondazione IRCCS Ca' Granda Maggiore Hospital, Università degli Studi di Milano, Milan, Italy

PIETRO LAMPERTICO, MD, PhD
1st Division of Gastroenterology, "A.M. e A. Migliavacca" Center for the Study of Liver Disease, Fondazione IRCCS Cà Granda Ospedale Maggiore Policlinico, Università degli Studi di Milano, Milano, Italy

YUN-FAN LIAW, MD
Professor, Liver Research Unit, Chang Gung Memorial Hospital, Chang Gung University College of Medicine, Taipei, Taiwan

GIAMPAOLO MANGIA, MD
1st Division of Gastroenterology, "A.M. e A. Migliavacca" Center for the Study of Liver Disease, Fondazione IRCCS Cà Granda Ospedale Maggiore Policlinico, Università degli Studi di Milano, Milano, Italy

PATRICK MARCELLIN, MD, PhD
Professor of Medicine, University Paris Diderot, Department of Hepatology, Hôpital Beaujon, Clichy, France

MICHELLE MARTINOT-PEIGNOUX, MD
INSERM U773/CRB3, Université Paris-Diderot, Paris, France

EVA POVEDA, PhD
Department of Infectious Diseases, Hospital Carlos III, Madrid, Spain

MARIO RIZZETTO, MD
Division of Gastroenterology, University of Torino, Torino, Italy

BRUNO ROCHE, MD
AP-HP Hôpital Paul Brousse, Centre Hépato-Biliaire; INSERM, Research Unit 785; Univ Paris-Sud, Health Research Unit 785, Villejuif, France

DIDIER SAMUEL, MD, PhD
AP-HP Hôpital Paul Brousse, Centre Hépato-Biliaire; INSERM, Research Unit 785; Univ Paris-Sud, Health Research Unit 785, Villejuif, France

VINCENT SORIANO, MD, PhD
Department of Infectious Diseases, Hospital Carlos III, Madrid, Spain

MAURO VIGANÒ, MD, PhD
Hepatology Division, Ospedale San Giuseppe, Università degli Studi di Milano, Milan, Italy

EUGENIA VISPO, MD
Department of Infectious Diseases, Hospital Carlos III, Madrid, Spain

Contents

The hepatitis B virus (HBV) plays a dominant role in the 749,000 new cases and 692,000 deaths related to hepatocellular carcinoma (HCC) that are estimated to occur each year worldwide. Chronic infection with HBV is responsible for 60% of HCCs in Asia and Africa and at least 20% of the tumors in Europe, Japan, and the United States. This article discusses the pathogenic role of HBV and the risk of HCC. Tumors almost invariably develop in the context of chronic hepatitis or cirrhosis, which makes early diagnosis the only practical approach to improve prognosis. The treatment options are also discussed.

There is a growing interest in serum HBsAg quantification (qHbsAg). HBsAg titers are negatively correlated with liver fibrosis in HBeAg(+) patients. In HBeAg(−) HBsAg level <1000 IU/mL and HBV-DNA titer <2000 IU/mL accurately identify inactive carriers. During PEG-IFN treatment qHBsAg identifies patients with no benefit from therapy at week 12, allowing stopping or switched *"week 12 stopping rule."* During nucleos(t)ide analogues the role of qHBsAg need to be clarified. In clinical practice qHBsAg is a simple and reproducible tool that may be used in association with HBV-DNA to classify patients during the natural history of HBV and to monitor therapy.

Chronic hepatitis B virus (HBV) infection is a dynamic state of interactions between HBV, the hepatocytes, and the patient's immune system. HBV replication is the key driving force for the HBV-related immune clearance events that determine the outcomes. The extended immune clearance phase is associated with liver disease progression, including development of cirrhosis and hepatocellular carcinoma (HCC). Thus, the primary aim of therapy is to eliminate or permanently suppress HBV to reduce hepatitis activity and thereby reduce the risk or slow the progression of liver disease.

Persistent viral eradication or suppression through a defined course of Pegylated-interferon (PegIFN) or the administration of a long-term potent nucleot(s)ide analogues (NUCs) can impact positively the natural course of HBV infection by preventing disease progression. Despite the higher rates of off-therapy response achieved with PegIFN compared with NUC, its benefits are restricted to a subgroup of patients only. To increase the rates of patients who may benefit from PegIFN treatment, minimizing the adverse events, careful patient selections based on baseline features and on treatment HBsAg kinetics for individual treatment optimization are required.

Chronic hepatitis B virus (HBV) infection, affecting approximately 350 to 400 million people worldwide, is associated with significant morbidity and mortality. Chronic hepatitis B remains a public health issue despite marked progress in public intervention programs. Individuals with chronic HBV infection have an increased risk for cirrhosis, decompensated liver disease, and hepatocellular carcinoma. The availability of safe and effective vaccines has reduced the burden of diseases. The choice of appropriate pharmacotherapy is critical in altering the course of the infection and reducing the costs associated with the management of chronic hepatitis B.

Antiviral therapy using newer nucleos(t)ide analogs with lower resistance rates could suppress hepatitis B virus (HBV) replication, improve liver function in patients with compensated or decompensated cirrhosis, delay or obviate liver transplantation in some patients, and reduce the risk of HBV recurrence. Some form of HBV prophylaxis needs to be continued indefinitely posttransplant. However, in patients with a low-risk of HBV recurrence it is possible to discontinue hepatitis B immunoglobulins and maintain long-term nucleos(t)ide analog therapy. Currently, treatment of posttransplantation hepatitis B is a less important clinical problem than it was historically because effective antiviral therapies exist to rescue patients who failed initial prophylaxis.

Hepatitis D is returning to western Europe through immigration. The clinical presentation recapitulates the typical features of a florid hepatitis D. Hepatitis D is also being rediscovered in the developing world and in the United States. Hepatitis D virus (HDV) remains endemic in many countries and efforts are underway to map the infection at local levels and improve the medical alert to hepatitis D. In the United States it is generally thought that HDV has gone and hepatitis D is no longer a problem. Awareness of hepatitis D in the country has recently been revived.

Vincent Soriano, Eva Poveda, Eugenia Vispo, and Pablo Barreiro

Chronic hepatitis B virus (HBV) infection is common in HIV-positive individuals. Although HBV vaccination is mandatory for HIV-positive individuals with negative-HBV markers, lower rates of protection are achieved.
HIV infection accelerates the course of liver disease caused by chronic
HBV infection, leading to end-stage hepatic illness and increasing the
risk of hepatocellular carcinoma. Anti-HBV active agents, especially tenofovir, improve outcomes. Lamivudine alone should be limited to patients
with low serum HBV-DNA levels, since selection of drug resistance often
compromises long-term benefits, leads to cross-resistance with other
antivirals, and favors the potential emergence of HBV-vaccine escape
mutants.

CLINICS IN LIVER DISEASE

RELATED INTEREST

Gastrointestinal Endoscopy Clinics of North America, April 2013, (Vol. 23, No. 2)
Endoscopic Approach to the Patient with Biliary Tract Disease
Jacques Van Dam, MD, PhD, *Editor*

NOW AVAILABLE FOR YOUR iPhone and iPad

Preface

An Update in the Management of Chronic Hepatitis B

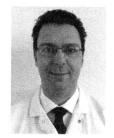 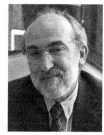

Tarik Asselah, MD, PhD   Patrick Marcellin, MD, PhD
Editors

This issue of *Clinics in Liver Disease* is dedicated to chronic hepatitis B, with several reviews from outstanding international experts.

Chronic hepatitis B virus (HBV) infection, affecting approximately 350 to 400 million people worldwide, is associated with significant morbidity and mortality. Individuals with chronic HBV infection have an increased risk for cirrhosis, decompensated liver disease, and hepatocellular carcinoma. The availability of safe and effective vaccines has reduced the burden of diseases. However, HBV infection continues to be the cause of considerable morbidity and mortality. In these last 10 years, advances have been made in leading several therapeutic options, including pegylated-interferon-α and nucleoside and nucleotide analogs. Both entecavir and tenofovir have demonstrated considerable efficacy.

In this issue are reported results of treatment of chronic hepatitis B with pegylated interferon and with nucleoside and nucleotide analogs (entecavir and tenofovir). Of particular interest is the long-term outcome of patients receiving the most potent available antiviral drugs and also their long-term impact. The clinical significance of HBsAg quantification is discussed as well as its role as a new tool for predicting response to therapy. Furthermore, an outstanding review on HBV infection and hepatocellular carcinoma is provided. The optimal management of special populations and difficult situations is extensively discussed: HIV-HBV co-infection and cirrhosis; and HBV-related decompensated cirrhosis and liver-transplanted patients. A review on hepatitis D is included. Finally, the ultimate goal of this issue is to review the most

Clin Liver Dis 17 (2013) ix–x
http://dx.doi.org/10.1016/j.cld.2013.05.009
1089-3261/13/$ – see front matter © 2013 Published by Elsevier Inc.

liver.theclinics.com

current knowledge and discuss therapeutic applications with the most experienced experts to provide optimal management of patients with HBV.

Tarik Asselah, MD, PhD
Service d'Hépatologie et Inserm U773-CRB3
University Paris-Diderot
Department of Hepatology, Hôpital Beaujon
100 Boulevard Général Leclerc
92110 Clichy, France

Patrick Marcellin, MD, PhD
Service d'Hépatologie et Inserm U773-CRB3
University Paris-Diderot
Department of Hepatology, Hôpital Beaujon
100 Boulevard Général Leclerc
92110 Clichy, France

E-mail addresses:
tarik.asselah@bjn.aphp.fr (T. Asselah)
patrick.marcellin@bjn.aphp.fr (P. Marcellin)

HBV Infection and Hepatocellular Carcinoma

Massimo Iavarone, MD, Massimo Colombo, MD*

KEYWORDS

- Hepatitis B • Hepatocellular carcinoma • Interferon • Nucleos(t)ide analogues
- Surveillance

KEY POINTS

- Safe and effective sterilizing vaccine against hepatitis B virus (HBV) has already been proved to actively antagonize hepatocellular carcinoma (HCC) in the juvenile population of endemic regions.
- Another preventive measure against HCC is screening/surveillance of patients with HBV with abdominal ultrasonography, which aims to improve HCC treatment through early diagnosis, the only practical approach to reduce liver-related mortality.
- It is still unclear whether permanent suppression of HBV by nucleos(t)ide analogs may also translate into a reduced risk of HCC in carriers, while preventing liver-related death from clinical decompensation.

INTRODUCTION

After the discovery of the serologic marker of the hepatitis B virus (HBV) in 1967, a wealth of epidemiologic data began to accumulate that progressively highlighted the role of HBV in hepatocellular carcinoma (HCC) worldwide. However, it was not until 1981, long before the basic mechanisms of HBV-related carcinogenesis could be fully elucidated by molecular studies of cell biology, that HBV was unequivocally linked to HCC through the landmark study by Palmer Beasley in Taiwan.[1] After prospective follow-up of more than 19,000 male state employees who were covered by a nationwide program of medical care and had their health status records traceable to death, it was found that virtually every case of HCC occurred in chronic carriers of HBV in whom the relative risk of developing HCC was ultimately greater than 200-fold that in uninfected controls. Since a similar link between HBV and HCC was subsequently demonstrated in the black population in South Africa, another endemic area for liver tumors, it was clear that HCC in those geographic areas could only be efficiently

1st Division of Gastroenterology, A.M. & A. Migliavacca Center for Liver Disease, Fondazione IRCCS Ca' Granda Maggiore Hospital, Università degli Studi di Milano, Via F. Sforza 35, Milan 20122, Italy
* Corresponding author. 1st Division of Gastroenterology, Fondazione IRCCS Ca' Granda Maggiore Hospital, Università degli Studi di Milano, Via F. Sforza 35, Milan 20122, Italy.
E-mail address: massimo.colombo@unimi.it

Clin Liver Dis 17 (2013) 375–397
http://dx.doi.org/10.1016/j.cld.2013.05.002
1089-3261/13/$ – see front matter © 2013 Elsevier Inc. All rights reserved.

liver.theclinics.com

fought by interrupting the perinatal transmission of HBV, which was the dominant modality of infection in the general population. The advent of a safe and effective sterilizing vaccine served the purpose, allowing us to dream about the possible eradication of hepatitis B. The battle started in Taiwan with a vaccination campaign for neonates of infected mothers, a program that was subsequently extended to mass vaccination of all neonates. As a result, the rates of chronic hepatitis B among teens decreased remarkably (from 10% to less than 1%) leading to a 50% drop in the rates of mortality from HCC in the same population.[2] Although the battle to prevent HBV-related HCC is running successfully to the point that more than 320 million neonates have been targeted thus far, substantial improvements have also been made in the management of patients who already have HCC, since standardization of the policies for the diagnosis and treatment of the tumor and the underlying hepatitis B. Currently, the guidelines for the management of HCC have been updated and optimized as a result of multidisciplinary contributions from experts in the scientific communities in the United States, Europe, and Asia Pacific to generate recommendations based on evidence and with the aim of developing cost-effective personalized therapies.[3–5]

EPIDEMIOLOGY

HBV is the dominant risk factor for HCC, which represents more than 90% of all liver cancers and each year accounts for 749,000 new cases and 692,000 HCC-related deaths.[6] Because of geographic variations in the incidence of hepatitis B, the fraction of HCC attributable to HBV varies significantly in various continents, representing less than 20% of all cases of HCC in the United States and up to 65% in China and Far East; Europe is divided into a low risk (18%) area (west and north Europe) and a high risk (51%) area (east and south Europe). However, the role of HBV in HCC may be greater than that depicted by seroepidemiologic studies, as suggested by the existence of hepatitis B surface antigen (HBsAg) seronegative individuals who may harbor subclinical infection with HBV in the liver as both free and integrated forms of HBV-DNA (**Fig. 1**).[7,8] Although the potential of occult infection to spread to the uninfected population is questioned, there is circumstantial evidence that occult HBV infection may have clinical consequences because it may cause deterioration of preexisting liver disease and reactivate to severe hepatitis B after exposure to immunosuppressive regimens.[9] As the pattern of HBV infection is changing as a result of the mass vaccination of newborns and risk groups against HBV, a decline in the infection rates among the general population has been demonstrated in endemic areas, whereas the spread of HBV is on the increase in research-rich countries like the United States and northern Europe as a consequence of increased population exposure to parenteral risks.[10]

RISK FACTORS

Virus-related, host-related, dietary, and lifestyle factors are associated with an increased risk of HCC in patients who are chronically infected by HBV. Increasing age and male gender, both reflecting increased exposure to HBV, have long been known to enhance the risk for HCC. More recently, evidence has emerged that gender disparity in HCC risk may also reflect protection against this tumor by estrogen via a complex path involving hepatocyte nuclear factor-4α.[11] Hepatitis severity and coinfection with such hepatropic viruses as hepatitis D virus and hepatitis C virus (HCV), or human immunodeficiency virus have been found to boost the HCC risk during chronic infection with HBV. Alcohol abuse, which itself is a relevant risk factor for

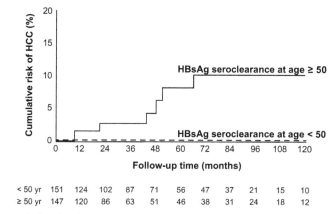

Fig. 1. Cumulative risk for development of HCC in patients with HBsAg seroclearance aged <50 years and ≥50 years. (*Data from* Yuen MF, Wong DK, Sablon E, et al. HBsAg seroclearance in chronic hepatitis B in the Chinese: virological, histologic, and clinical aspects. Hepatology 2004;39:1694–701; and Yuen MF, Wong DK, Fung J, et al. HBsAg seroclearance in chronic hepatitis B in Asian patients: replicative level and risk of hepatocellular carcinoma. Gastroenterology 2008;135:1192–9.)

HCC, plays a synergistic role by more than doubling the carcinogenic risk of HBV.[12] In Asia and Africa, dietary aflatoxin is another relevant contributor to HCC of regional importance; it is associated with increased risk of tumors in HBV-infected persons exposed to food contaminated by *Aspergillum flavus*.[13] Tobacco smoking is also associated with an increased risk of HCC in patients with HBV-related cirrhosis, with evidence of a quantitative relationship between smoking and cancer risk. Important epidemiologic aspects of HBV-related HCC that may have clinical relevance include younger age at presentation compared with HCC cases related to alcohol, nonalcoholic steatohepatitis, and HCV, the absence of cirrhosis in one-third of patients with HCC, and the correlation between HCC risk, HBV genotype, HBV genomic mutations, and serum levels of HBV replication[7,8]; the latter established the rationale for starting antiviral therapy in HBV carriers with trivial hepatic lesions. Prolonged antiviral therapy in patients with HBV has resulted in a paradoxic effect of reducing the risk of HCC in noncirrhotic patients by preventing progression to cirrhosis and reducing the rates of anticipated liver mortality due to clinical decompensation, leading to an increase in the rates of HCC-related mortality.

In the Far East more than in the West, studies of family clusters provided evidence for the existence of a family-based susceptibility to HCC. Undoubtedly, genetic host factors play an important role in the development of HCC during HBV infection, which may have important clinical applications. The most common form of genetic variation between individuals is single nucleotide polymorphisms (SNPs), which are a variation in the base at a particular nucleotide locus; a common SNP is defined as having a minor allele frequency of at least 5%. Initial studies were designed with a candidate gene approach, in which a limited number of biologically plausible SNPs was tested.

The starting hypothesis is that a given variant in a specific gene involved in a pathway that influences HCC development can sufficiently alter either protein function or expression, and result in the modulation of cancer risk. Another approach to study genetic factors is through genome-wide association studies (GWAS), hypothesis free by definition, and comparison of the allele/genotype frequency of common variants between cases and unaffected controls and testing 100,000s of tag SNPs, reflecting common genetic variations across the entire human genome. To reach GWAS significance ($P = .05$/number of SNPs tested), a P value in the order of less than 10^{-8} is typically required.[14] Susceptible genetic variants for HBV-related HCC have been sought by many genetic association studies with a case-control, retrospective, or single-center design.[15] Most studies focused on selected Asiatic populations thereby minimizing ethnicity diversity and calling for external validation in populations of different ancestry before effectively translating the results to clinical practice. The loss of heterozygosity on the KIF1B locus, a common genetic lesion in a broad range of human cancers, has been identified as a susceptibility marker for HCC in patients with chronic hepatitis B.[16] Variations at chromosome 8p12 seem to be associated with HCC in patients with HBV and the risk-associated 8p12 SNPs or haplotypes might have an interacting effect on the DLC1 locus (Deleted in Liver Cancer 1), which becomes more susceptible to deletion or chromosomal loss.[17] In a retrospective case-control analysis using a candidate gene approach in patients with chronic hepatitis B, other genes involved in immune and carcinogenesis processes were found to have a significant association with HCC development; for example, cytotoxic T-lymphocyte antigen 4 gene, the promoter region of the MCM7 gene and enhancer II (EnhII), basal core promoter (BCP), and precore regions of HBV (**Table 1**).[18–20] Unfortunately, the SNPs identified so far only partly explain the overall variability in HCC susceptibility. Because they carry a low risk ratio for HCC development, these genes have mostly been assessed in well-selected patients from whom HCC tissue was obtained after surgical resection (selection bias), therefore not permitting prediction at both the individual and population levels.

PATHOGENESIS

HCC stems from multistep accumulation of genetic and epigenetic changes conferring unlimited self-sufficient growth and resistance to physiologic homeostatic

Table 1
Genetic associations with HCC in patients with chronic HBV infection

Author, Year	Study Design	Time	Patients		SNP Locus	Strength (OR)
Zhang et al,[16] 2010	GWAS	N	CHB CHB-HCC	1790 2317	KIF1b	0.6
Chan,[17] 2011	GWAS	3.0	CHB CHB-HCC	825 595	DLC1	1.3
Gu et al,[18] 2010	Candidate gene	1.0	HBV negative CHB CHB-HCC	419 209 375	CTLA-4	1.7
Chou et al,[19] 2008	Candidate gene	14	CHB CHB-HCC	316 154	EnhII/BCP region	2.2–4.7
Liu et al,[20] 2012	Candidate gene	5.0	HBV negative CHB CHB-HCC	1344 1344 1300	MCM7	1.2

Abbreviations: CHB, chronic hepatitis B; GWAS, genome-wide association study; HCC, hepatocellular carcinoma; OR, adds ratio.

mechanisms.[21] The long latency of tumor development after primary infection with HBV indicates the existence of indirect oncogenic pathways based on multiple cooperative mechanisms that integrate the direct genetic or epigenetic effects of the virus. Although this explains why HCC may also arise during the pre-cirrhotic phase of chronic hepatitis B, the oncogenic mechanisms of HBV remain enigmatic. HBV frequently gets integrated into the host genome causing DNA rearrangement and enhanced mutagenesis; active cell inflammation and proliferation, fostering the accumulation of genetic and epigenetic alterations, may act synergistically by both increasing the opportunity for such events to occur and promoting their selection. Integration of HBV DNA into host chromosomes almost invariably occurs in infected patients leading to insertional mutagenesis of cancer-related genes and chromosomal instability, whereas certain viral proteins like the HBx transactivator, participate as cofactors in the oncogenetic process. One important cellular event accounting for the sequential acquisition of premalignant and malignant characteristics is persistent liver cell inflammation associated with oxidative stress, which provokes repeated cycles of apoptosis, necrosis, and compensatory regeneration. HCC may result from faulty regulation of liver cell senescence, which is involved in tumor immune surveillance, senescence surveillance of premalignant hepatocytes representing an important barrier against tumor development.[22] Hepatic fibrosis may also be relevant to HCC pathogenesis as suggested by high-grade dysplastic nodules in fibrotic livers that are the immediate precursors of HCC,[23,24] as well as chromosomal aberrations and epigenetic modifications such as DNA methylation leading to the silencing of tumor suppressor genes that have been described in cirrhosis.[25,26] Oncogenic mutations affecting mostly the p53 and β-catenin genes are seen at the tumoral stage.[27] Although genetic instability plays a crucial role in tumor initiation and progression, many studies have demonstrated genetic heterogeneity of HCC, with significant differences depending on the etiology; in particular, tumors related to the HBV cluster in subclasses characterized by high genetic instability, notably with aberrations at chromosomes 4q, 13q, 16p, 16q, 17p.[28,29] Increased genetic instability may be triggered by specific HBV features including integration of viral DNA into host chromosomes and HBx protein activity. Integration of HBV DNA sequences in the host genome occurs because early stages of acute infections and multiple integrations have been detected in chronic hepatitis tissues. Clonal integrated HBV sequences have been seen in about 80% of HBV-related HCCs.[30] The notion that HBV integrates randomly into human chromosomes has been challenged by recent data supporting viral insertion in the induction of the first genetic hit in the carcinogenesis process and the identification of target genes in hepatocarcinogenesis, as shown earlier for HBV insertions into the retinoic acid receptor b and cyclin A2 genes.[31,32] Recent studies have shown that HBx interferes with the normal control of cell cycle progression, through its ability to bind different cellular partners and to activate transcription as well as various signaling cascades.[33] Moreover, HBx has been implicated in deregulation of the mitotic phase and in induction of chromosomal instability.

NATURAL HISTORY OF THE TUMOR

HCC is a stepwise process usually but not necessarily starting from the cirrhosis stage and dysplastic regenerative nodules.[34] Both conditions are characterized by increased cell division and stepwise accumulation of genetic changes necessary for cell transformation, including telomerase shortening with accumulation of senescent hepatocytes, limitation of regenerative reserve, and induction of chromosomal instability. The heterogeneity of the natural history of HCC largely reflects the multiplicity of the pathogenic molecular mechanisms involved in carcinogenesis, such as enhanced liver cell proliferation, leading to loss of replicative competition and selection of malignant clones, promoted also by alterations in the microenvironment and the macroenvironment.[35] Among the genetic alterations that are closely associated with clinical features of HCC, defining the relevant pattern of HBV hepatocarcinogenesis, chromosome instability stands as the hallmark of HBV-related HCC in contrast with chromosome stability, which is mostly related to alcohol and HCV.[29] By analysis of transcriptive genotype/phenotype correlations, 6 main subgroups (G1 to G6) of HCC have been identified that are associated with clinical and genetic alterations.[36] G1 and G2 identify HBV-infected patients, as well as tumors with genetic instability that are strikingly distinct from other HCCs in terms of molecular signature. Subgroup G1 includes HBV-related tumors from younger patients, frequently seen in Africa and sharing the same characteristics as the hepatoblastoma type of HCC described by Lee and colleagues[37] at the National Institutes of Health. This genetic classification of HCC was recently confirmed by a meta-analysis[38] supporting previous clinical and pathologic studies showing that HCV-related tumors are more often multicentric than HBV-related tumors.[39,40] From a clinical point of view, another important hallmark of HBV-related tumors is younger age at presentation and lower rates of cirrhosis compared with HCV-related tumors. In a large study in Italy,[41] cirrhosis was detected in 73% of HCV-infected patients compared with 44% of HBV-infected patients. Irrespective of the severity of the underling liver disease, the risk of HCC in HBV carriers is greater in Asia than in the West, likely as a consequence of earlier exposure to HBV and to dietary carcinogens such as aflatoxin.[13]

Although HCC is first detected as a single, slowly growing nodule,[34] the tumor size when detected does not predict the course of the disease in all cases; the median time for doubling of the volume for a small HCC ranges from 1 to 20 months with significant differences in the growth rates for each nodule even in cirrhotic livers harboring multiple HCCs.[42] Although the tumor is a clinically indolent disease during the early phases of growth, advanced HCC may present with painful hepatomegaly, jaundice, or systemic symptoms. In at least one-third of patients, HCC is first detected as a multinodular disease, more commonly in patients with multiple causative factors such as viral hepatitis plus alcohol than in those with a single causative factor.[43] The wide differences in the growth pattern of HCC may have clinical implications, thereby influencing the choice and outcome of treatments. In general, slowly expanding tumors have a more favorable prognosis than fast-growing, replacing type tumors.[44] Prognostication may be difficult in HCCs that have constant rates of growth during follow-up; others either have a declining growth rate in the late phases of follow-up or, after an initial phase of resting, increase in volume exponentially.[45] This great diversity of tumor growth patterns explains why prognostication in patients with HCC can be obtained more reliably by combining tumor number and size, portal vein invasion by the tumor, and clinical data such as symptoms and liver impairment (**Table 2**).

The presence of vessel invasion by the tumor has important clinical implications because it heralds a risk of tumor recurrence for patients with macroscopic venous invasion.[46]

EARLY DIAGNOSIS

Most patients with HCC are identified with advanced disease that almost invariably prevents application of curative treatments. Conversely, early diagnosis through surveillance improves both the applicability and outcome of HCC therapy; the recall policy, that is, the type of tests applied to confirm HCC, varies according to the size

Table 2
The Barcelona Clinic Liver Cancer (BCLC) staging classification for HCC

BCLC Stage	Performance Status	Tumor Volume, Number, and Invasiveness	Child-Pugh
0 Very early	0	$\leq$2 cm vaguely nodular	A
A Early	0	Single <5 cm or 3 nodes <3 cm each	A and B
B Intermediate	0	Large/multinodular	A and B
C Advanced	1–2	Vascular invasion and/or extrahepatic spread	A and B
D End stage	3–4	Any of the above	C

Modified from Forner A, Reig ME, de Lope CR, et al. Current strategy for staging and treatment: the BCLC update and future prospects. Semin Liver Dis 2010;30:61–74; with permission.

of a liver nodule (**Fig. 2**). A nodule less than 10 mm in diameter is difficult to diagnose by contrast computed tomography (CT) scan, magnetic resonance imaging (MRI), or by echo-guided liver biopsy. In this situation, a recall policy is better served by enhanced follow-up with ultrasonography (US) every 3 months with the aim of detecting any increase in size or pattern that may guide further investigations with radiology or liver biopsy.[3,4] Nodules greater than 10 mm in diameter, which represent 80% of tumors detected during surveillance, can be diagnosed by CT or MRI whenever the specific pattern of intense contrast uptake during the arterial phase (wash-in) is followed by contrast wash-out during the venous/delayed phase.[3,4] In Europe and the United States, contrast-enhanced US is not recommended as the sole diagnostic imaging technique, because it does not accurately distinguish intrahepatic cholangiocarcinoma from HCC.[47] The American Association for the Study of Liver Disease (AASLD) algorithm for investigating nodules greater than 10 mm in diameter endorses the sequential use of a single imaging technique between CT and MRI as long as it demonstrates the radiological hallmark of HCC (contrast wash-in in the arterial phase followed by wash-out in the portal venous and/or delayed phases). The use of a single technique in a sequential study has eased surveillance for HCC, because it has reduced the need for fine-needle biopsy procedures to diagnose HCC, without affecting the sensitivity and specificity rates of the recall policy.[48–50] It should be recalled, however, that these noninvasive diagnostic criteria are only valid for investigation of screen-detected lesions in cirrhosis or chronic hepatitis B that may not yet have fully developed cirrhosis.[3,4,51] The serum alfafetoprotein (AFP) assay is no longer considered for screening (and diagnosis) because of poor accuracy and the lack of a standardized recall policy[3,4]; the biannual combination of US + AFP has no added value compared with US alone for the early diagnosis of HCC.[52]

The Barcelona Clinic Liver Cancer (BCLC) classification, which is endorsed by both AASLD and the European Association for the Study of the Liver (EASL), comprises 2 categories of early tumors: very early and early HCC. The former is a tumor less than 2 cm in diameter in a patient with perfectly compensated cirrhosis (Child Pugh A) that lacks arterial hypervascularization at contrast imaging, thereby requiring histologic confirmation (in situ or stage 0 HCC). The second category is a single tumor less than 5 cm in diameter or up to 3 tumors each smaller than 3 cm arising in a patient with Child Pugh A or B cirrhosis (stage A HCC) (see **Table 2**).[3,4] The end point of an early diagnosis being achieved in a minority of patients with HCC, most clustering in the developed world, since surveillance involves more than simply a screening test; it must involve a program in which tests, recall policies, and quality control procedures

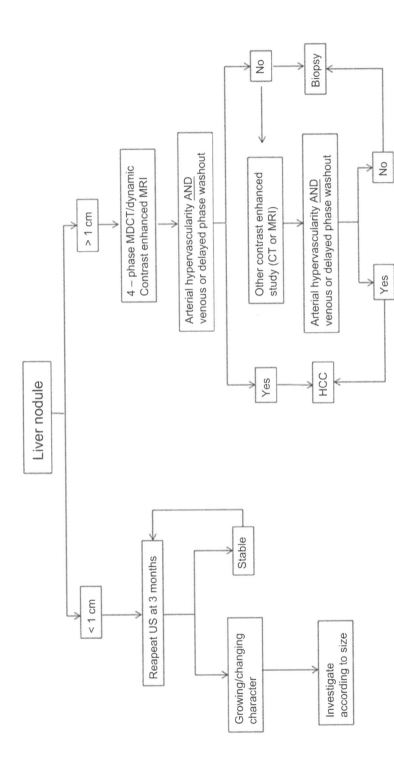

Fig. 2. 2010 AASLD algorithm for investigation of small nodules found on screening in patients with cirrhosis. (*Modified from* Bruix J, Sherman M, American Association for the Study of Liver Diseases. Management of hepatocellular carcinoma: an update. Hepatology 2011;53:1020–2; with permission.)

are standardized, with significant economic consequences. Because HCC develops in the background of well-recognized environmental risk factors, chronic liver disease above all, and the screening test adopted (US) is user friendly, accurate, and acceptable to the population, surveillance has gained popularity even in the absence of robust evidence that it reduces liver-related mortality. There is only 1 randomized controlled study supporting screening for liver cancer in patients with chronic liver disease, which was conducted in the Shanghai area, but it was flawed by potential biases in patient selection, treatment, and study conduct (**Table 3**).[53] Thus, the real support for screening for liver cancer in patients with chronic liver disease comes from numerous retrospective surveys that have reported striking differences in response to therapy between screened populations and patients with incidental tumors. However, these studies were biased by anticipated diagnosis (lead time bias) and improved access to treatments, which do not necessarily translate into reduced liver-related mortality. In view of the chasm between efficacy and effectiveness, an argument was made by the National Cancer Institute against dissemination of HCC screening in the United States, to some extent echoing the reluctance of many physicians to accept screening as a standard of care for HCC, as emerged recently in a population-based study in the United States in which only 6.6% of 3903 Medicare patients with HCC were shown to receive regular surveillance before diagnosis.[54] The finding of a low rate of screening uptake (12%) was replicated among veterans infected with HCV with cirrhosis.[55] In those surveys gastroenterologists, hepatologists, or physicians with an academic affiliation were more likely to perform surveillance than practitioners involved in community-based practices, which suggests that barriers to screening such as limited or outdated knowledge and not only a lack of financial incentives, limited access to appropriate testing and treatment, ultimately working against effectiveness of screening.

THE COST-USEFULNESS RATIO OF SCREENING

AASLD considers screening worthwhile in selected populations such patients with HCV with 1.5% or more incidence of HCC, HBV patients with more than 0.2% incidence, and, in general, patients with cirrhosis with more than 2.5% incidence. Although the benefits are intuitive, the economic consequences of surveillance

Table 3		
A RCT of population-based screening for HCC: the importance of early diagnosis for improving liver-related mortality		
Findings	**Screened Group**	**Control Group**
Patients × year	38,444	41,077
HCC Occurrence		
Cases	86	67
Early cancer	39	0
Total incidence (per 100,000)	223.7	163.1
Rate ratio (95% CI)	1.37 (0.99, 1.89)	Reference
Deaths from HCC		
Deaths	32	54
Total mortality (per 100,000)	83.2	131.5
Rate ratio (95% CI)	0.63 (0.41, 0.98)	Reference

strategies are poorly appreciated because of the lack of randomized trials evaluating moderators of treatment outcome such as compliance, heterogeneity of liver disease, and treatment effectiveness, which, in addition to tumor incidence, affect the cost-usefulness ratio of surveillance. In the absence of randomized controlled trials (RCTs), the cost-effectiveness of surveillance has been analyzed by Markov modeling, but within the framework of epidemiologic and interventional assumptions that do not necessarily reflect real-life practice. Further attenuating the credibility of modeling is the a priori decision to measure cost-usefulness ratios at less than US$ 50,000 for quality-adjusted life year saved, an assumption that may conflict with policies of equitability while being influenced by the economic trends worldwide. In principle, strengthening prediction in individual patients is expected to improve cost-effectiveness ratios of screening, but the benefits of approaches such as stratification of pretreatment patients by clinical, histologic, and genetic scores remain uncertain.[56,57] Given that the goal of screening is to reduce disease-specific mortality, certain restrictions such as exclusion of patients with severe comorbidities who do not fit the criteria for curative therapies are also warranted. Whether screening should be restricted to older individuals who would not have significant benefit if diagnosed with an HCC is also under debate.

TUMOR PROGNOSTICATION

The outcome of HCC largely depends on patient suitability for curative treatments, which in turn are greatly influenced by tumor staging combining tumor characteristics, performance status, and liver function. The size and number of HCC nodes are the best clinical surrogates predicting tumor dedifferentiation and vascular invasion, which are independent predictors of shortened survival in patients undergoing liver resection.[34] The BCLC staging classification[58] comprises 5 stages that select the best candidates for the best therapies available, that is, from very early tumor (stage 0) and early tumor (stage A) including asymptomatic patients with small tumors suitable for radical therapies to more advanced tumor stages up to untreatable disease (see **Table 2**). In referral centers, approximately one-third of patients present with an early stage tumor that is fit for radical treatment after proper selection. Hepatic resection, liver transplantation, and percutaneous interstitial treatments may provide 5-year survival rates between 50% and 70%. Patients with a tumor larger than 5 cm or more than 3 nodules each less than 3 cm in size, with compensated liver disease lacking vascular invasion or extrahepatic spread of the tumor, have an expected spontaneous survival of 50% at 3 years (intermediate stage of BCLC). Similar patients with more deteriorated liver function and/or vascular invasion and/or extrahepatic spread of the tumor have advanced tumor disease, with a dismal prognosis of less than 10% survival at 3 year (stage C of BCLC). End-stage HCC includes terminal patients, including Child-Pugh C patients whose survival does not exceed 6 months.

In recent years, other staging systems have been proposed including the CLIP staging system, the Chinese University Prognostic Index,[59] the modified TNM,[60] a French scoring system,[61] and a German scoring system.[62] Because staging scores developed thus far reflect differences in the demographic features of the patients seen locally, expertise, and treatment algorithms adopted in different centers, is it worth attempting to reach consensus on a single model for staging HCC? From a clinical point of view, it seems mandatory that prognostication of liver cancer should always incorporate treatment-dependent variables.[63] In several studies, BCLC proved to be superior to other scores in the prognostication of patients with HCC.[64,65]

TREATMENT ALGORITHMS

Hepatic resection, orthotropic liver transplantation (LT), and percutaneous tumor ablation of carefully selected patients are potentially curative treatments of HCC (**Fig. 3**). Conversely, palliative treatments include transhepatic arterial chemoembolization (TACE) and systemic therapy with sorafenib (see **Fig. 3**).[3,4] Patients with HCC in a normal liver or mild/moderate chronic hepatitis are ideal candidates for liver resection. However, due to the frequent association of HCC with cirrhosis, hepatic resection is only applicable in a minority of patients with a small tumor and well-compensated liver function. Patients with poorly compensated cirrhosis are definitively contraindicated for hepatic resection, because the operation may precipitate liver failure, whereas they may be eligible for LT. Pretreatment patient assessment is best served by CT scan or MRI, a chest CT scan, and a bone scan. The presence of portal invasion by the tumor or extrahepatic localization of tumor indicates a bleak prognosis, and precludes curative interventions. The general conditions of the patient as reflected by the performance status (PS) score are also essential parts of pretreatment patient evaluation.[51,66]

Patients with a Noncirrhotic Liver

Noncirrhotic patients account for less than 10% of all patients with HCC in the West compared with 40% of patients in Asia, where the leading risk factor, HBV, may cause HCC during the precirrhotic phase of the infection.[5] Those patients are ideal candidates for liver resection, but their survival largely depends on tumor volume at diagnosis. Patients with a tumor developing in a normal liver who are identified outside screening programs, and often present with a large, symptomatic tumor, have the worst prognosis.

Patients with Cirrhosis

Very early/early HCC

Very early HCC (BCLC stage 0) is a single tumor (<20 mm) without vascular invasion or satellites developing in patients with a good health status (PS 0) and well-preserved liver function (Child-Pugh A). Approximately 10% of all patients in the West and up to 30% in Japan are currently diagnosed in this stage as a consequence of the widespread implementation of surveillance programs. Pathologically, these tumors appear as vaguely nodular, without local invasiveness by tumor cells (carcinoma in situ), a situation that may translate to 5-year survival rates greater than 70% after resection or percutaneous local ablation.

Early HCC (BCLC stage A) is a single tumor less than 50 mm in size (tumors >50 mm carry a high risk of vascular invasion and satellites) or 3 nodules each less than 30 mm, PS 0, and Child-Pugh A/B. The 5-year survival in accurately selected patients ranges between 50% and 70% after hepatic resection, LT, or percutaneous local ablation. Although very early tumors are best indicated for local ablative therapies, resection is the best option for patients with a single tumor of any size, although the risk of vascular invasion and dissemination by tumor cells causing postoperative recurrence of the tumor increases with tumor size. However, in the few patients in whom HCC may grow slowly to reach more than 50 mm in size without causing liver invasion or satellite nodules, an effective and safe hepatic resection is feasible with a moderate risk of tumor recurrence as in patients with smaller tumors. After hepatic resection of an HCC 50 mm or less in a compensated patient, the 5-year survival rates approach 50%, but with a 70% risk of tumor recurrence. In more than half of the patients undergoing radical resection, tumor recurs during the first 18 months as a consequence of

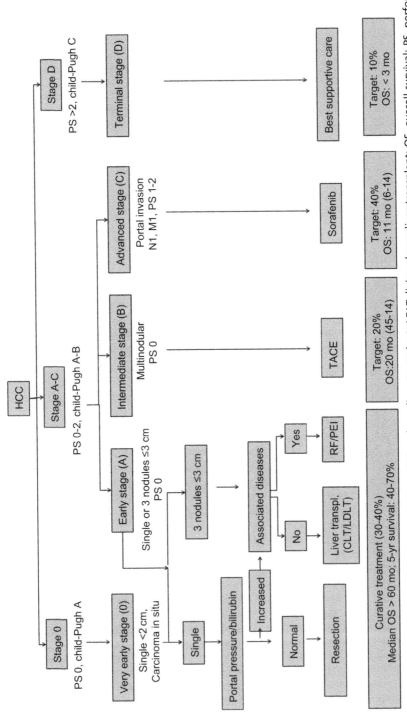

Fig. 3. BCLC staging system and treatment strategy. CLT, cadaver liver transplant; LDLT, living donor liver transplant; OS, overall survival; PS, performance status. (*Adapted from* European Association for the Study of the Liver, European Organisation for Research and Treatment of Cancer. EASL-EORTC clinical practice guidelines: management of hepatocellular carcinoma. J Hepatol 2012;56:908–43; with permission.)

preoperative and postoperative tumor cell dissemination[67]; in 30% of resected patients, tumor recurs between 2 and 5 years after the operation as a consequence of de novo primary tumors developing in the cirrhotic liver. Although the most powerful predictors of early postoperative recurrence are microvascular invasion by the tumor, tumor cell grading, and satellite nodules,[68] no effective neoadjuvant or adjuvant treatments are available to reduce the risk of recurrence. Hepatic resection is also associated with an increased risk of postoperative (3 months) fatal liver failure caused by reduced functional reserve of the remnant liver, an adverse event that can be predicted by preoperative assessment of portal hypertension. The risk of liver failure is greater for patients with a portocaval gradient more than 10 mm Hg, such as patients with esophageal varices and patients with a serum bilirubin level greater than 1 mg/dL, in whom hepatic resection may result in a 5-year rate of survival of 25%, compared with the rate of 75% for patients with none of these adverse predictors.[69]

HCC is the only solid cancer for which organ transplantation is an established treatment modality. Theoretically, LT has the advantage of simultaneous eradication of both tumor and underlying hepatitis B; the efficacy of the treatment is only marginally influenced by the degree of liver impairment. The Milan criteria for patient selection based on a single HCC of 5 cm or less or up to 3 nodules, each 3 cm or less in size, without vascular invasion or extrahepatic spread, resulted in a fair balance between a 4-year survival rate of 75% and a limited risk (8%) of tumor recurrence.[46] After external validation in several liver centers worldwide, the Milan criteria are now the benchmark for patient selection in both the United States and Europe. Since the success of LT in patients with HCC is challenged by the shortage of donors leading to increased waiting times and risk of tumor progression, the effectiveness of LT needs to be evaluated in terms of intention-to-treat analysis.[70] Whenever the waiting time exceeds 6 months, bridge treatments with tumor ablation and TACE aimed at delaying disease progression, are currently offered, whereas hepatic resection is the first choice for patients with favorable predictors of survival leaving LT for patients with adverse predictors of response to resection. Although access to LT has been successfully improved by strategies based on split liver and living related liver donors, the strategy of expanding listing criteria beyond Milan is not endorsed by all centers, and is highly debated in terms of cost-effectiveness, particularly in regions with a limited donor supply. Using the up-to-seven criteria, which allow for a total tumor diameter of 12 cm compared with a maximum of 9 cm for Milan and 8 cm for the University of California San Francisco criteria, a continuous range of survival probabilities, rather than a dichotomous in or out basis for patient selection, is provided.[71,72] However, the 5-year survival of patients who were transplanted within the up-to-seven criteria but exceeded the Milan criteria was only 54%.

Percutaneous tumor ablation is a consolidated treatment option for patients with an early HCC who do not fit the criteria for surgery[73]; radiofrequency ablation (RFA) together with percutaneous ethanol injection (PEI) are the most widely adopted therapeutic approaches in nonresectable small tumors. Both percutaneous techniques achieve complete tumor necrosis in almost 100% of patients with nodules of 20 mm or less, whereas RFA is more effective than PEI in tumors of 30 mm due to better control of the periphery of the tumor nodule. However, both techniques lose efficacy in tumors larger than 30 mm because of the presence of satellites to the point that tumor ablation with RFA or PEI is no longer recommended for nodules greater than 30 to 40 mm.[74] In properly selected patients with compensated cirrhosis, percutaneous tumor ablation may confer 5-year survival rates of 50% to 75%, thus mimicking the satisfactory rates of efficacy of hepatic resection as a first-line therapeutic option. Despite several RCTs comparing the outcome of percutaneous ablation and resection in early HCC, there is no definite demonstration of the clinical superiority of one procedure over the other. The main reasons for discrepancies between studies were inadequate sample size, treatment allocation, and trial conduct. Novel techniques such as microwaves or electroporation are under evaluation to treat early HCC. Adjuvant approaches with interferon and cytotoxic anticancer agents failed to demonstrate activity against HCC. An RCT (STORM [Sorafenib as adjuvant Treatment in the prevention Of Recurrence of hepatocellular carcinoMa]) is in progress to assess the efficacy of adjuvant therapy with sorafenib to improve disease-free survival after hepatic resection or percutaneous ablation of tumors at risk of recurrence.

Intermediate HCC (BCLC stage B)

BCLC stage B involves patients exceeding the Milan criteria, but without portal vein invasion or extrahepatic spread of the tumor. TACE, combining the injection of cytotoxic drugs such as oxaliplatin and doxorubicin, with embolic obstruction of the arterial blood supply of the tumor, caused more than 50% of patients to have an objective response, which translated into an improved average survival from 16 to 22 months.[75] One step forward was the development drug-eluting bead (DEB) TACE based on the injection of microspheres to increase the local concentration of the cytotoxic drugs. This approach allows standardization of the TACE procedure and reduces drug-related adverse events caused by absorption of cytotoxic drugs.[76] The ideal candidates for TACE are compensated patients with an asymptomatic, large/multifocal HCC restricted to the liver that is not amenable to curative treatments. TACE should be delivered in more than 1 course either as protocol treatment or on demand, whenever the tumor nodules become revascularized after each successful procedure. To delay tumor revascularization, an antiangiogenic agent such as sorafenib is being assessed in combination with DEB TACE. Radioembolization with yttrium 90–labeled microspheres is an attractive option for patients with intermediate or advanced HCC, including patients with portal invasion by the tumor who are contraindicated for DEB TACE.[77] However, no controlled data on survival of patients treated with yttrium 90 are available.

Advanced HCC (BCLC stage C)

Patients with symptomatic tumors (PS 1–2), macrovascular invasion, or tumor spread in lymph nodes, lung, and skeleton have an expected median survival of 6 months (25% at 1 year). Although interferon, hormones, and cytotoxic anticancer drugs failed to demonstrate any activity against HCC in controlled trials,[3,4,51] targeted therapy with sorafenib is now the standard of care for BCLC stage C patients with clinically compensated cirrhosis, because it can attenuate tumor progression and invasiveness. Sorafenib, through its activity against RAF signaling as well as vascular endothelial growth factor, platelet-derived growth factor, and c-kit, is the only agent that has been proved to improve survival in patients with advanced HCC. In a registration study in patients with HCC, sorafenib prolonged patient survival by approximately 3 months, causing a 31% decrease in the relative risk of death.[78] Similar survival benefits have also been obtained for HBV-related tumors in a study conducted in the Asia Pacific region[79]; a limited number of adverse events occurred that were usually manageable. Sorafenib is the standard of care not only for compensated patients with advanced HCC (BCLC stage C) but also for compensated patients with a tumor not responding to locoregional therapies. No second-line drugs for nonresponders to sorafenib are available as yet (see www.clinicaltrial.gov).

End-stage HCC (BCLC stage D)

Patients with end-stage disease who have a very poor performance status (PS 3–4), resulting in a median survival of 3 to 4 months (11% at 1 year) should receive the best supportive care.

Assessment of tumor response

Although patient survival is the end point in cancer therapy, objective tumor responses are necessary surrogates for predicting treatment efficacy in registration trials and monitoring treatment effectiveness in practice. The Response Evaluation Criteria In Solid Tumors (RECIST) based on morphometric changes in the tumor volume[80] do not accurately evaluate HCC response to therapy as they do not take arterial vascularity of the tumor nodule into account. Paradoxically, nodules treated with invasive procedures may be enlarged at radiology as a consequence of edema accompanying tumor tissue necrosis. Modified RECIST evaluates a response to both invasive and drug-related therapy for HCC, based on the viable tumor cells identified by contrast imaging.[81]

PRIMARY PREVENTION

Because HCC develops in the context of readily identifiable environmental risk factors such as HBV, successful primary prevention strategies are possible. Screening of donated blood, widespread use of disposable medical devices, and vaccination against HBV have led to a significant decrease in the rates of new cases of hepatitis B in developed countries. In 1984, Taiwan started a program of universal vaccination of newborns to mothers who were HBV carriers that was subsequently extended to all newborns, and preschool and school children and teenagers, with a significant impact on the rate of HBsAg carriers among children, which decreased from 9.8% in 1984 to 0.7% in 1999. In parallel, a decrease in HCC incidence from 0.70 per 100,000 children to 0.36 was noted; a few children (3.4%) among those who had not received hepatitis B immunoglobulin prophylaxis at birth had vaccine failure, therefore remained exposed to the risk of maternal transmission of HBV.[2] To date, universal HBV vaccination of newborns has been introduced in more than 150 countries worldwide.

Given the ability of anti-HBV regimens to determine cirrhosis regression in a large number of cases, there is a biological plausibility for sustained viral replication suppression with nucleos(t)ide analogs (NUC) in patients with chronic hepatitis B to reduce the risk of neoplastic transformation of the liver. Prevention of HCC in patients with chronic hepatitis B with a maintained virological response to therapy is far from being convincingly demonstrated especially because this dramatic and life-threatening complication occurs in most patients many decades after viral infections and many years after diagnosis of hepatitis. Thus, a study designed to assess primary prevention of HCC through chemotherapy in HBV populations should therefore not only follow up patients for improbably long periods of time after treatment complications but also exclude patients for whom treatment failed from any form of retreatment while maintaining them on clinical observation, a fact that is obviously impossible and unethical.

The scrutiny of trials of anti-HBV therapy was a hint to investigate chemoprevention of HCC in patients with chronic hepatitis B, yet it provided difficult to interpret the information. All therapeutic trials designed to assess antiviral efficacy of anti-HBV regimens adopted surrogate end points and therefore were underpowered to capture hard end points of hepatitis B including HCC. In the interferon setting, patient enrollment was skewed toward less severe hepatitis to improve patient compliance, which resulted in selection bias and a diluted risk of HCC in the study population, as well as different duration and accuracy of follow-up between patients with a virological response to interferon versus nonresponders. In most studies, patients were not stratified before treatment by such relevant predictors of HCC as age and sex, disease severity, lifestyle, and comorbidities, which compromises comparison between studies. Thus, caution needs to be exerted in the interpretation of the systematic review of meta-analysis on the effect of interferon versus no treatment on the development of HBV-related HCC. Three studies[82–84] show prevention of HCC by interferon, but with exceptions between studies; for example, one study reported no benefit in noncirrhotic patients,[85] whereas another study demonstrated prevention of HCC by interferon in non-European cohorts only. In contrast, 3 meta-analyses showed no benefits of interferon therapy, because HCC occurred at the same rates in treated and untreated patients with chronic hepatitis B. However, 1 study[86] included patients with compensated cirrhosis only[85–87]; the benefits of a virological response are easier to evaluate in these patients because they are the closest to developing hepatitis-related complications such as decompensation and cancer (**Table 4**).

In the setting of NUC therapy, several studies have shown that patients with HBV who achieved a virological response to lamivudine in some cases still developed HCC, which was the only complication arising in virological responders (see **Table 1**).[86] In a systematic review of studies of NUC treatment of patients with HBV, it was clearly defined that HCC was prevented in patients with chronic hepatitis but not in those with cirrhosis, and, in general, in patients who could not achieve complete virological suppression. This was confirmed by a recent cohort study from Greece in which cirrhotic patients on long-term lamivudine were shown to remain at risk of developing liver cancer (**Fig. 4**). Given that all these studies enrolled patients treated with lamivudine or rescued with adefovir, an obvious question is whether more potent anti-HBV drugs, such as entecavir and tenofovir, might actually confer an advantage in terms of HCC prevention in responders with cirrhosis. However, this was not the case in a multicenter study in Italy where patients with compensated cirrhosis who had persistently undetectable serum HBV DNA during 5 years of

Table 4
Meta-analyses on the effect of interferon versus no treatment on the development of HBV-related HCC

Authors, Year	No. of Studies	No. Treated vs Controls	Relative Risk/Risk Difference[a] (95% CI)	P	Comments
Sung et al,[82] 2008	12	1292 vs 1458	0.66 (0.48–0.89)	.006	No effect in noncirrhotic patients
Yang et al,[83] 2009	11	1006 vs 1076	0.59 (0.43–0.81)	.001	Normal alanine aminotransferase level excluded
Miyake et al,[84] 2009	8	553 vs 750	5.0%[a] (9.4–0.5)	.028	Effect not shown in Europeans
Cammà et al,[85] 2001	7	853 vs 652	4.8%[a] (0.11–0.015)	NS	All cirrhotic patients
Zhang et al,[86] 2011	2	176 vs 171	0.23 (0.05–1.04)	NS	
Jin et al,[87] 2011	9	1291 vs 1048	0.274 (0.059–1.031)	NS	

[a] Risk difference.

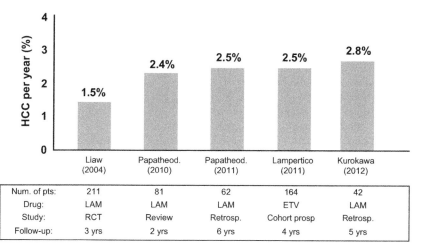

Fig. 4. HCC rates in NUC-naive cirrhotic patients with long-term response to NUC. ETV, entecavir; LAM, lamivudine. (*Adapted from* Aghemo A, Lampertico P, Colombo M. Assessing long-term treatment efficacy in chronic hepatitis B and C: between evidence and common sense. J Hepatol 2012;57:1326–35; with permission.)

entecavir monotherapy showed an annual rate of neoplastic transformation of the liver of approximately 2.5%, thus mimicking the HCC rates in untreated HBeAg-negative patients in Europe (**Fig. 5**).[88] Persistence of HCC risk in cirrhotics responding to NUC therapy may be the consequence of an extended survival provided by NUCs preventing clinical decompensation, as was found in the Italian multicenter study. On the other hand, HBV-related liver carcinogenesis is likely to be promoted by cellular events that are established early during chronic infection with HBV, independently of the onset of cirrhosis. This would explain why NUCs can determine regression of cirrhosis, protection from clinical decompensation and variceal bleeding, but not from HCC development.

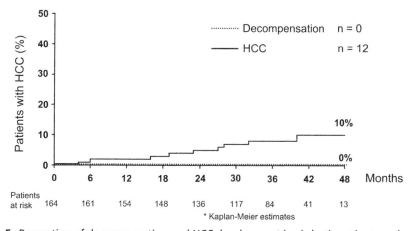

Fig. 5. Prevention of decompensation and HCC development in cirrhotic patients under entecavir monotherapy. (*Adapted from* Lampertico P, Vigano M, Soffredini R, et al. Entecavir monotherapy for nuc-naive chronic hepatitis B patients from field practice: high efficacy and favorable safety profile over 3 years. Hepatology 2011;54(Suppl 1):Abstract 1436.)

SUMMARY

Although abundant epidemiologic, clinical, and experimental data link HCC to HBV infection, particularly when acquired early in life, the cascade of pathogenic events leading to HBV-induced liver carcinogenesis has not completely been worked out. It is clear that the pathogenic paradigm of HCC in patients with chronic hepatitis B often implies a direct quantitative relationship between tumor risk and HBV replication, but HCC developing in patients with either subclinical or occult infection with HBV paves the way for alternative and complementary interpretations of the role of this virus in HCC; it may act as a carcinogen to the liver through functions that are unrelated to active replication. In the 1980s, the development of a safe and effective sterilizing vaccine against HBV was a major breakthrough in medicine that has already been proved to actively antagonize HCC in the juvenile population of the endemic regions where mass vaccination of neonates was implemented. In the next decades, it is expected to definitively benefit the adult population in more than 150 nations who participated in the GAVI program. Another, yet less implemented, preventive measure against HCC is screening/surveillance of HBV patients using abdominal US, which aims to improve HCC treatment through early diagnosis, the only practical approach to reduce liver-related mortality in carriers. Despite intense retrospective scrutiny of therapeutic trials with anti-HBV regimens, particularly with NUC, it is still unclear whether permanent suppression of HBV may also translate into a reduced risk of HCC in carriers, a question that may have important implications because of the ability of most of these treatments to prevent liver-related death from clinical decompensation. The paradox of increased longevity of cirrhotic patients after prevention of decompensation with NUC therapy resulting in an enhanced risk of developing HCC has led to a remarkable shift in the indications for LT in patients with HBV from clinical decompensation to HCC in a compensated liver, a scenario that resulted in substantial survival benefits compared with the hepatitis C situation, mainly due to prevention of graft reinfection. This is not a trivial point, because in a scenario of equitable resources competing in favor of distributive justice, differences in posttransplant survival between patients HBV and HCV might open the door for the argument that HCC is a criterion for prioritization to LT.

REFERENCES

1. Beasley RP, Hwang LY, Lin CC, et al. Hepatocellular carcinoma and hepatitis B virus. A prospective study of 22 707 men in Taiwan. Lancet 1981;2:1129–33.
2. Chang MH, Chen CJ, Lai MS, et al. Universal hepatitis B vaccination in Taiwan and the incidence of hepatocellular carcinoma in children. Taiwan Childhood Hepatoma Study Group. N Engl J Med 1997;336(26):1855–9.
3. Bruix J, Sherman M. Management of hepatocellular carcinoma: an update. Hepatology 2011;53:1020–2.
4. European Association for the Study of the Liver, European Organisation for Research and Treatment of Cancer. EASL-EORTC clinical practice guidelines: management of hepatocellular carcinoma. J Hepatol 2012;56(4):908–43.
5. Omata M, Lesmana LA, Tateishi R, et al. Asian Pacific Association for the Study of the Liver consensus recommendations on hepatocellular carcinoma. Hepatol Int 2010;4:439–74.
6. Perz JF, Armstrong GL, Farrington LA, et al. The contributions of hepatitis B virus and hepatitis C virus infections to cirrhosis and primary liver cancer worldwide. J Hepatol 2006;45:529–38.

7. Di Bisceglie AM. Hepatitis B and hepatocellular carcinoma. Hepatology 2009; 49:S56–60.
8. Chen CJ, Yang HI, Su J, et al, REVEAL-HBV Study Group. Risk of hepatocellular carcinoma across a biological gradient of serum hepatitis B virus DNA level. JAMA 2006;295(1):65–73.
9. Raimondo G, Pollicino T, Squadrito G. What is the clinical impact of occult hepatitis B virus infection. Lancet 2005;365:638–40.
10. Kew MC. Epidemiology of chronic hepatitis B virus infection, hepatocellular carcinoma, and hepatitis B virus-induced hepatocellular carcinoma. Pathol Biol 2010;58(4):273–7.
11. Wang SH, Yeh SH, Lin WH, et al. Estrogen receptor α represses transcription of HBV genes via interaction with hepatocyte nuclear factor 4α. Gastroenterology 2012;142(4):989–98.
12. Donato F, Tagger A, Gelatti U, et al. Alcohol and hepatocellular carcinoma: the effect of lifetime intake and hepatitis virus infections in men and women. Am J Epidemiol 2002;155:323–31.
13. Ming L, Thorgeirsson S, Gail MH, et al. Dominant role of hepatitis B virus and cofactor role of aflatoxin in hepatocarcinogenesis in Qidong, China. Hepatology 2002;36:1214–20.
14. Pearson TA, Manolio TA. How to interpret a genome-wide association study. JAMA 2008;299:1335–44.
15. Nahon P, Zucman-Rossi J. Single nucleotide polymorphisms and risk of hepato-cellular carcinoma in cirrhosis. J Hepatol 2012;57(3):663–74.
16. Zhang H, Zhai Y, Hu Z, et al. Genome-wide association study identifies 1p36.22 as a new susceptibility locus for hepatocellular carcinoma in chronic hepatitis B virus carriers. Nat Genet 2010;42(9):755–8.
17. Chan LK, Ko FC, Sze KM, et al. Nuclear-targeted deleted in liver cancer 1 (DLC1) is less efficient in exerting its tumor suppressive activity both in vitro and in vivo. PLoS One 2011;6(9):e25547.
18. Gu X, Qi P, Zhou F, et al. +49G > A polymorphism in the cytotoxic T-lymphocyte antigen-4 gene increases susceptibility to hepatitis B-related hepatocellular carcinoma in a male Chinese population. Hum Immunol 2010;71(1):83–7.
19. Chou YC, Yu MW, Wu CF, et al. Temporal relationship between hepatitis B virus enhancer II/basal core promoter sequence variation and risk of hepatocellular carcinoma. Gut 2008;57(1):91–7.
20. Liu Y, Zhang Y, Wen J, et al. A genetic variant in the promoter region of miR-106b-25 cluster and risk of HBV infection and hepatocellular carcinoma. PLoS One 2012;7(2):e32230.
21. Llovet JM, Burroughs A, Bruix J. Hepatocellular carcinoma. Lancet 2003;362: 1907–17.
22. Kang TW, Yevsa T, Woller N, et al. Senescence surveillance of pre-malignant hepatocytes limits liver cancer development. Nature 2011;479:547–51.
23. Friedman SL. Mechanisms of hepatic fibrogenesis. Gastroenterology 2008;134: 1655–69.
24. Lee JM, Wong CM, Ng IO. Hepatitis B virus-associated multistep hepatocarcino-genesis: a stepwise increase in allelic alterations. Cancer Res 2008;68:5988–96.
25. Kanai Y. Genome-wide DNA methylation profiles in precancerous conditions and cancers. Cancer Sci 2010;101:36–45.
26. Um TH, Kim H, Oh BK, et al. Aberrant CpG island hypermethylation in dysplastic nodules and early HCC of hepatitis B virus-related human multistep hepatocar-cinogenesis. J Hepatol 2011;54:939–47.

27. Imbeaud S, Ladeiro Y, Zucman-Rossi J. Identification of novel oncogenes and tumor suppressors in hepatocellular carcinoma. Semin Liver Dis 2010;30:75–86.

28. Marchio A, Pineau P, Meddeb M, et al. Distinct chromosomal abnormality pattern in primary liver cancer of non-B, non-C patients. Oncogene 2000;19:3733–8.

29. Laurent-Puig P, Legoix P, Bluteau O, et al. Genetic alterations associated with hepatocellular carcinomas define distinct pathways of hepatocarcinogenesis. Gastroenterology 2001;120:1763–73.

30. Brechot C. Pathogenesis of hepatitis B virus-related hepatocellular carcinoma: old and new paradigms. Gastroenterology 2004;127:S56–61.

31. Dejean A, Bougueleret L, Grzeschik KH, et al. Hepatitis B virus DNA integration in a sequence homologous to v-erbA and steroid receptor genes in a hepatocellular carcinoma. Nature 1986;322:70–2.

32. Wang J, Chenivesse X, Henglein B, et al. Hepatitis B virus integration in a cyclin A gene in a human hepatocellular carcinoma. Nature 1990;343:555–7.

33. Benhenda S, Cougot D, Buendia MA, et al. Hepatitis B virus X protein molecular functions and its role in virus life cycle and pathogenesis. Adv Cancer Res 2009; 103:75–109.

34. Bruix J, Sherman M, Llovet JM, et al, for the EASL Panel of Experts on HCC. Clinical management of hepatocellular carcinoma. Conclusions of the Barcelona – 2000 EASL Conference. J Hepatol 2001;35:421–30.

35. El-Serag HB, Rudolph R. Hepatocellular carcinoma: epidemiology and molecular carcinogenesis. Gastroenterology 2007;132:2557–76.

36. Boyault S, Rickman DS, de Reynies A, et al. Transcriptome classification of HCC is related to gene alterations and to new therapeutic targets. Hepatology 2007; 45:42–52.

37. Lee JS, Chu IS, Heo J, et al. Classification and prediction of survival in hepatocellular carcinoma by gene expression profiling. Hepatology 2004;40:667–76.

38. Hoshida Y, Nijman SM, Kobayashi M, et al. Integrative transcriptome analysis reveals common molecular subclasses of human hepatocellular carcinoma. Cancer Res 2009;69(18):7385–92.

39. Shiratori Y, Shina S, Imamura M, et al. Characteristic difference of hepatocellular carcinoma between hepatitis B- and C- viral infection in Japan. Hepatology 1995;22:1027–33.

40. Miyagawa S, Kawasaki S, Makuuchi M. Comparison of the characteristics of hepatocellular carcinoma between hepatitis B and C viral infection: tumor multicentricity in cirrhotic liver with hepatitis C. Hepatology 1996;24:307–10.

41. Stroffolini T, Andreone P, Andriulli A, et al. Characteristics of hepatocellular carcinoma in Italy. J Hepatol 1998;29:944–52.

42. Colombo M, de Franchis R, Del Ninno E, et al. Hepatocellular carcinoma in Italian patients with cirrhosis. N Engl J Med 1991;325:675–80.

43. Fasani P, Sangiovanni A, De Fazio C, et al. High prevalence of multinodular hepatocellular carcinoma in patients with cirrhosis attributable to multiple risk factors. Hepatology 1999;29:1704–7.

44. Anthony PP. Primary carcinoma of the liver: a study of 282 cases in Ugandan Africans. J Pathol 1973;110(1):37–48.

45. Okazaki N, Yoshino M, Yoshida T, et al. Evaluation of the prognosis for small hepatocellular carcinoma based on tumor volume doubling time. A preliminary report. Cancer 1989;63(11):2207–10.

46. Mazzaferro V, Regalia E, Doci R, et al. Liver transplantation for the treatment of small hepatocellular carcinomas in patients with cirrhosis. N Engl J Med 1996; 334:693–9.

47. Vilana R, Forner A, Bianchi L, et al. Intrahepatic peripheral cholangiocarcinoma in cirrhosis patients may display a vascular pattern similar to hepatocellular carcinoma on contrast-enhanced ultrasound. Hepatology 2010;51(6): 2020–9.

48. Forner A, Vilana R, Ayuso C, et al. Diagnosis of hepatic nodules 20 mm or smaller in cirrhosis: prospective validation of the noninvasive diagnostic criteria for hepatocellular carcinoma. Hepatology 2008;47(1):97–104.

49. Sangiovanni A, Manini MA, Iavarone M, et al. The diagnostic and economic impact of contrast imaging techniques in the diagnosis of small hepatocellular carcinoma in cirrhosis. Gut 2010;59:638–44.

50. Khalili K, Kim TK, Jang HJ, et al. Optimization of imaging diagnosis of 1-2 cm hepatocellular carcinoma: an analysis of diagnostic performance and resource utilization. J Hepatol 2011;54(4):723–8.

51. Forner A, Llovet JM, Bruix J. Hepatocellular carcinoma. Lancet 2012;379(9822): 1245–55.

52. Singal A, Volk ML, Waljee A, et al. Meta-analysis: surveillance with ultrasound for early-stage hepatocellular carcinoma in patients with cirrhosis. Aliment Pharmacol Ther 2009;30:37–47.

53. Zhang BH, Yang BH, Tang ZY. Randomized controlled trial of screening for hepatocellular carcinoma. J Cancer Res Clin Oncol 2004;130:417–22.

54. Davila JA, Morgan RO, Richardson PA, et al. Use of surveillance for hepatocellular carcinoma among patients with cirrhosis in the United States. Hepatology 2010;52:132–41.

55. Davila JA, Henderson L, Kramer J, et al. Utilization of surveillance for hepatocellular carcinoma among hepatitis C virus–infected veterans in the United States. Ann Intern Med 2011;154:85–93.

56. Velazquez RF, Rodríguez M, Navascues CA, et al. Prospective analysis of risk factors for hepatocellular carcinoma in patients with liver cirrhosis. Hepatology 2003;37(3):520–7.

57. Ganne-Carrié N, Chastang C, Chapel F, et al. Predictive score for the development of hepatocellular carcinoma and additional value of liver large cell dysplasia in Western patients with cirrhosis. Hepatology 1996;23:1112–8.

58. Llovet JM, Brú C, Bruix J. Prognosis of hepatocellular carcinoma: the BCLC staging classification. Semin Liver Dis 1999;19(3):329–38.

59. Leung TW, Tang AM, Zee B, et al. Construction of the Chinese University Prognostic Index for hepatocellular carcinoma and comparison with the TNM staging system, the Okuda staging system, and the Cancer of the Liver Italian Program staging system: a study based on 926 patients. Cancer 2002;94(6): 1760–9.

60. Henderson JM, Sherman M, Tavill A, et al. AHPBA/AJCC consensus conference on staging of hepatocellular carcinoma: consensus statement. HPB (Oxford) 2003;5(4):243–50.

61. Chevret S, Trinchet JC, Mathieu D, et al. A new prognostic classification for predicting survival in patients with hepatocellular carcinoma. Groupe d'Etude et de Traitement du Carcinome Hepatocellulaire. J Hepatol 1999;31(1):133–41.

62. Rabe C, Lenz M, Schmitz V, et al. An independent evaluation of modern prognostic scores in a central European cohort of 120 patients with hepatocellular carcinoma. Eur J Gastroenterol Hepatol 2003;15:1305–15.

63. Sangiovanni A, Del Ninno E, Fasani P, et al. Increased survival of cirrhotic patients with a hepatocellular carcinoma detected during surveillance. Gastroenterology 2004;12:1005–14.

64. Marrero JA, Fontana RJ, Barrat A, et al. Prognosis of hepatocellular carcinoma: comparison of 7 staging systems in an American cohort. Hepatology 2005; 41(4):707–16.

65. Cillo U, Vitale A, Grigoletto F, et al. Prospective validation of the Barcelona Clinic Liver Cancer staging system. J Hepatol 2006;44(4):723–31.

66. Sorensen JB, Klee M, Palshof T, et al. Performance status assessment in cancer patients. An inter-observer variability study. Br J Cancer 1993;67:773–5.

67. Imamura H, Matsuyama Y, Tanaka E, et al. Risk factors contributing to early and late phase intrahepatic recurrence of hepatocellular carcinoma after hepatectomy. J Hepatol 2003;38(2):200–7.

68. Nagasue N, Uchida M, Makino Y, et al. Incidence and factors associated with intrahepatic recurrence following resection of hepatocellular carcinoma. Gastroenterology 1993;105:488–94.

69. Bruix J, Castells A, Bosch J, et al. Surgical resection of hepatocellular carcinoma in cirrhotic patients: prognostic value of preoperative portal pressure. Gastroenterology 1996;111:1018–22.

70. Llovet JM, Fuster J, Bruix J. Intention-to-treat analysis of surgical treatment for early hepatocellular carcinoma: resection versus transplantation. Hepatology 1999;30:1434–40.

71. Mazzaferro V, Llovet JM, Miceli R, et al, Metroticket Investigator Study Group. Predicting survival after liver transplantation in patients with hepatocellular carcinoma beyond the Milan criteria: a retrospective, exploratory analysis. Lancet Oncol 2009;10(1):35–43.

72. Yao FY, Ferrell L, Bass NM, et al. Liver transplantation for hepatocellular carcinoma: expansion of the tumor size limits does not adversely impact survival. Hepatology 2001;33:1394–403.

73. Lencioni R. Loco-regional treatment of hepatocellular carcinoma. Hepatology 2010;52:762–73.

74. Germani G, Pleguezuelo M, Gurusamy K, et al. Clinical outcomes of radiofrequency ablation, percutaneous alcohol and acetic acid injection for hepatocellular carcinoma: a meta-analysis. J Hepatol 2010;52:380–8.

75. Llovet JM, Bruix J. Systematic review of randomized trials for unresectable hepatocellular carcinoma: chemoembolization improves survival. Hepatology 2003;37:429–42.

76. Lammer J, Malagari K, Vogl T, et al. Prospective randomized study of doxorubicin-eluting bead embolization in the treatment of hepatocellular carcinoma: results of the PRECISION V study. Cardiovasc Intervent Radiol 2010; 33:41–52.

77. Salem R, Lewandowski RJ, Mulcahy MF, et al. Radioembolization for hepatocellular carcinoma using Yttrium-90 microspheres: a comprehensive report of long-term outcomes. Gastroenterology 2010;138:52–64.

78. Llovet J, Ricci S, Mazzaferro V, et al. Sorafenib in advanced hepatocellular carcinoma. N Engl J Med 2008;359:378–90.

79. Cheng AL, Kang YK, Chen Z, et al. Efficacy and safety of sorafenib in patients in the Asia-Pacific region with advanced hepatocellular carcinoma: a phase III randomised, double-blind, placebo controlled trial. Lancet Oncol 2009;10: 25–34.

80. Therasse P, Arbuck SG, Eisenhauer EA, et al. New guidelines to evaluate the response to treatment in solid tumors. European Organization for Research and Treatment of Cancer, National Cancer Institute of the United States, National Cancer Institute of Canada. J Natl Cancer Inst 2000;92:205–16.

81. Lencioni R, Llovet JM. Modified RECIST (mRECIST) assessment for hepatocellular carcinoma. Semin Liver Dis 2010;30(1):52–60.
82. Sung JJ, Tsoi KK, Wong VW, et al. Meta-analysis: treatment of hepatitis B infection reduces risk of hepatocellular carcinoma. Aliment Pharmacol Ther 2008;28:1067–77.
83. Yang YF, Zhao W, Zhong YD, et al. Interferon therapy in chronic hepatitis B reduces progression to cirrhosis and hepatocellular carcinoma: a meta-analysis. J Viral Hepat 2009;16:265–71.
84. Miyake Y, Kobashi H, Yamamoto K. Meta-analysis: the effect of interferon on development of hepatocellular carcinoma in patients with chronic hepatitis B virus infection. J Gastroenterol 2009;44:470–5.
85. Cammà C, Giunta M, Andreone P, et al. Interferon and prevention of hepatocellular carcinoma in viral cirrhosis: an evidence-based approach. J Hepatol 2001;34:593–602.
86. Zhang CH, Xu GL, Jia WD, et al. Effects of interferon treatment on development and progression of hepatocellular carcinoma in patients with chronic virus infection: a meta-analysis of randomized controlled trials. Int J Cancer 2011;129:1254–64.
87. Jin H, Pan N, Mou Y, et al. Long-term effect of interferon treatment on the progression of chronic hepatitis B: Bayesian meta-analysis and meta-regression. Hepatol Res 2011;41:512–23.
88. Lampertico P, Soffredini R, Vigano M, et al. Entecavir treatment for NUC naïve, field practice patients with chronic hepatitis B: excellent viral suppression and safety profile over 5 years of treatment. Hepatology 2012;56(S1):370A.

HBsAg Quantification to Predict Natural History and Treatment Outcome in Chronic Hepatitis B Patients

Michelle Martinot-Peignoux, MD[a],*, Tarik Asselah, MD, PhD[a,b],
Patrick Marcellin, MD, PhD[a,b]

KEYWORDS

- Personalized medicine • Prediction • PEG-IFN • Analogues • HBV tools • Prognosis

KEY POINTS

- Serum hepatitis B surface antigen (HBsAg) level reflects the transcriptional activity of the covalently closed circular DNA in the liver.
- In hepatitis B e antigen (HBeAg)–positive chronic hepatitis B, HBsAg level is higher in the immune tolerance phase than the immune clearance phase.
- In HBeAg negative patients, combination of low hepatitis B virus (HBV) DNA and low HBsAg levels may predict inactive carrier status, low risk of hepatocellular carcinoma, and probability of HBsAg loss.
- HBsAg surrogate marker to predict peginterferon therapy outcome.
  - Absence of decline at week 12: prediction of non-response "stop therapy".
  - Any decline at week 24: prediction of response "continue therapy" 48 weeks.
- Although the HBsAg decline is slow with nucleos(t)ide analogue therapy, a rapid decline may predict future HBsAg seroclearance.

WHY QUANTIFY HEPATITIS B SURFACE ANTIGEN IN 2013

At baseline identification of

Inactive carriers
Severity of the liver disease
Probability of hepatocellular carcinoma (HCC)
Probability of hepatitis B surface antigen (HBsAg) loss

[a] INSERM U773/CRB3, Université Paris-Diderot, Paris, France; [b] Service d'Hépatologie, Hôpital Beaujon, 100 Boulevard du Général Leclerc, Clichy 92110, France
* Corresponding author. Hôpital Beaujon, 100 Boulevard du Général Leclerc, Clichy 92110, France.
E-mail address: michelle.martinot@inserm.fr

Clin Liver Dis 17 (2013) 399–412
http://dx.doi.org/10.1016/j.cld.2013.05.006
1089-3261/13/$ – see front matter © 2013 Elsevier Inc. All rights reserved.

HBsAg on treatment kinetics prediction of treatment outcome:

Pegylated interferon: stopping rule
  Increase treatment duration?
NUCs: stopping rule in hepatitis B e antigen (HBeAg)–positive patients?
  identification of patients with high probability of HBsAg loss.

The hepatitis B virus (HBV) is a small DNA virus. On entry into the cell, HBV sheds its protein coat, and the partially double-strand genome is transported into the nucleus of the hepatocyte, where it is transformed into a fully double-strand covalently closed circular DNA (cccDNA). The cccDNA resides in the nucleus of infected hepatocytes, where it acts as a template for transcription of the viral gene and recycles in the nucleus to renew the cccDNA pool.[1,2] Viral proteins of clinical importance include the envelope protein (HBsAg) whose synthesis during the HBV viral life cycle is complex. HBsAg production exceeds that required for virion assembly, and excess surface envelope proteins are covalently linked and secreted as empty non-infectious filamentous or spherical sub-viral particles.[3] These empty particles may co-exist with anti-HBs as part of circulating immune complexes.[4] Serum HBsAg is a result of the combination of these proteins (complete virion, filamentous or spherical sub-viral particles). HBsAg quantification measures all 3 forms of systemic HBsAg.

Several studies have shown the relationship between intrahepatic markers of HBV infection (cccDNA and integrated HVB DNA) and serum HBsAg.[3,5–7] Differences in HBsAg levels during the different phases of the disease reflect the distribution of cccDNA during the respective infection phases. HBsAg levels are higher in HBeAg positive (+) than in HBeAg negative (−) patients.[6–8]

CLINICAL APPLICATIONS

HBsAg seroconversion (loss of HBsAg and development of anti-HBs) is rarely observed during the natural course of chronic HBV infection. The annual incidence is 1% to 2% worldwide.[1] It is the ultimate goal of therapy. Recently, quantitative serum HBsAg assays have been developed,[9,10] and the importance of HBsAg quantification has been recognized as an important marker to monitor the natural history in chronic hepatitis and predict treatment outcome.[11–13] HBsAg levels decrease more in patients receiving interferon (IFN), an immune modulator, than in those receiving nucleos(t)ides analogues (NA), potent inhibitors of HBV DNA replication.[14]

HBSAG QUANTIFICATION

Several fully automated assays are commercially available. The assays most frequently used in Europe are the Cobas e411 HBsAg II assay (Roche Diagnostics GmbH Mannheim, Germany), the Architect HBsAg QT assay (Abbott, Chicago, IL USA), the ETI-MAK-1 assay (Diasorin, Turin Italy), and the Monolisa HBsAg ultra assay (Bio-Rad Laboratories Redmond, WA, USA). Results observed with both assays a very well correlated and closely in agreement across all HBV genotypes.

Studies have shown that serum HBsAg levels vary according to the different phases of HBV chronic infection. These observations emphasize that serum HBsAg levels reflect the interplay between the virus and the immune system providing complementary information on viral load. The interest in HBsAg quantification started with the possible observation of its association with the level of covalently closed circular (ccc) DNA, the template for viral replication inside the nuclei of hepatocytes. HBsAg has been shown to be a surrogate marker for cccDNA. Werlé–Lapostolle and colleagues[3] report a significant decrease in cccDNA and serum HBsAg and HBV

cutoff (3.85 $\log_{10}$ IU/mL) to identify moderate to severe fibrosis ($\geq$F2) in HBeAg(+) CHB patients infected with HBV genotypes B or C. This association was not observed in HBeAg($-$) patients.[28] There was no association between HBsAg titer and histologic grade found in either study.

HBsAg Level and Therapy

Interferon therapy

Only a small proportion of patients (3%–7%) experience HBsAg loss during 48 weeks of IFN-based therapy.[21] The efficacy of pegylated IFN (PEG-IFN) has been confirmed in 2 large pivotal studies.[29,30] The HBeAg seroconversion rate was observed in 32% in HBeAg(+) patients[29] and an HBV DNA less than 400 IU/mL in 19% in HBeAg($-$) patients.[30] In the early 1990s, HBsAg quantification was already considered to be a promising, simple, and inexpensive method to monitor viral replication in CHB patients who were receiving IFN treatment.[31] More recently, the availability of well-standardized commercial assays has renewed interest in the quantitative serum HBsAg as a biomarker for treatment response in CHB.[9,10]

HBeAg(+) patients

Current data[32–37] indicate that on treatment HBsAg quantification could help identify either patients with a high probability of sustained virological response (SVR) or nonresponders. In a study by Chan and colleagues,[32] SVR rates were 62% and 11% in patients with HBsAg less than or equal to 300 IU/mL and in those with HBsAg greater than 300 IU/mL at 24 weeks of therapy. The authors also showed that patients with a combined response of HBsAg less than or equal to 300 IU/mL and a decrease of greater than or equal to 1 $\log_{10}$ IU/mL at 24 weeks had higher SVR rates than those without the combined response (75% vs 15%), with a PPV and NPV of 75% and 85%, respectively. Tangkijvanich and colleagues[33] report that baseline HBsAg levels were lower in patients with HBeAg seroconversion at the end of therapy than in nonresponders. In the Neptune study,[35,37] the highest HBeAg seroconversion rates were observed in patients with HBsAg levels less than or equal to 1500 IU/mL at 12 or 24 weeks of therapy with a PPV of 57% or 54% and an NPV of 72% or 76%, respectively. These results confirm those of the phase III PEG-IFN alfa 2a trial.[34] Sonneveld and colleagues[36] showed that patients who received a combination of PEG-IFN plus lamivudine had a more pronounced on-treatment decrease in HBsAg patients than those who received PEG-IFN alone, although the former relapsed. The absence of decline at week 12 had an NPV of 97% for SVR and no chance of HBsAg loss. The study by Lau and colleagues[34] reported a lower NPV (82%) than the study by Sonneveld and colleagues. The discrepancies between the 2 studies[34,36] might be due to the different populations studied. Indeed, in the study by Sonneveld and colleagues, most of the patients had genotypes A and D, whereas the Lau study included genotypes B and C Asian patients. It is interesting to note that certain studies have reported a more significant decrease in HBsAg and more frequent HBsAg in patients with HBV genotype A who receive PEG-IFN.[38–40]

HBeAg(−) patients

The response rate to PEG-IFN is low (<20%) in HBeAg($-$) patients.[41–44] These patients are difficult to monitor. Indeed, most of them achieve undetectable serum HBV DNA at the end of therapy, but relapse when treatment is stopped.[30,43,44] Therefore, predictive factors of on-treatment response may help define more appropriate treatment strategies in certain patients. The most recent evidence suggests that HBsAg quantification is a worthwhile marker for monitoring PEG-IFN therapy (**Fig. 3**).[45–47]

Rijckborst and colleagues[43] reported that the combination of HBsAg and a decrease in HBV-DNA is the best predictor of an SVR in patients receiving

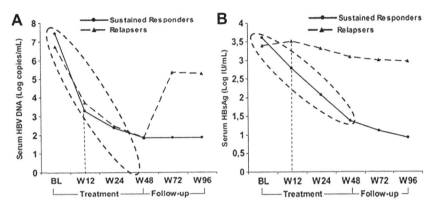

Fig. 3. Changes in serum HBV DNA (*A*) and HBsAg (*B*), during PEG-IFN therapy. Illustration of HBV DNA and HBsAg kinetics in sustained responder (*solid line*) and relapser (*dash line*) during peginterferon therapy. Serum HBV DNA was undetectable at the end of therapy (*A*) in both patients with SVR and with relapse. During therapy, HBsAg decreased (*B*) only in patients who developed SVR. (*Data from* Moucari R, Mackiewicz V, Lada O, et al. Early serum HBsAg drop: a strong predictor of sustained virological response to pegylated interferon alfa-2a in HBeAg-negative patients. Hepatology 2009;49:1151–7.)

PEG-IFN. A lack of decrease in HBsAg and a serum HBV DNA decline of less than 2 $\log_{10}$ IU/mL have an NPV of 100% for SVR. Another[45] study has shown that a serum HBsAg decrease of greater than or equal to 0.5 log IU/mL at week 12 had a high PPV of SVR (PPV 89%) and a lack of decrease of greater than or equal to 1 $\log_{10}$ IU/mL at week 24 had a high NPV of non-SVR (NPV 92%).

Studies have investigated end-treatment and post-treatment HBsAg titers to predict SVR and loss of HBsAg during post-treatment follow-up. In a cohort of 127 HBeAg(−) genotype D patients who received 48 weeks of PEG-IFN treatment, Brunetto and colleagues[46] showed that an on-treatment greater than or equal to 1 $\log_{10}$ IU/mL HBsAg decrease and an HBsAg level less than 10 IU/mL at the end of therapy were highly predictive for an SVR at the 24-week post-treatment follow-up and for HBsAg loss at the 3-year post-treatment follow-up. In this study, at the 3-year post-treatment follow-up an HBsAg loss was observed in 52% of the patients with an HBsAg less than 10 IU/mL at week 48 of treatment compared with only 2% of the patients with an HBsAg greater than 10 IU/mL at week 48. The authors did not find any association between serum HBV DNA response (<400 IU/mL) at the end of therapy and HBsAg loss. A French retrospective study[48] also reported that most of the patients who lost HBsAg during post-treatment follow-up had a greater than or equal to 1 $\log_{10}$ IU/mL decrease in HBsAg levels at the end of 48 weeks of IFN treatment followed by a steady decrease until seroclearance.

Week 12 stopping rule

Most studies report that the absence of a decrease in HBsAg or an HBV DNA decline of lower than 2 $\log_{10}$ after 12 to 24 weeks of a 48-week course of PEG-IFN is associated with an NPV of 84% to 100% for SVR (**Table 1**).[55] Rijckborst and colleagues[52] confirmed these results in patients in the Parc study[56] and performed external validation in the phase III registration study[28] and the PegBeLiver study,[56] both of which included patients with HBV genotypes A to D. There was an NPV greater than or equal to 95% for SVR in both validation studies in the absence of a decrease in HBsAg or a decline in HBV DNA less than 2 $\log_{10}$ IU/mL at week 12 of treatment. The authors

Table 1
SVR as predicted by serum HBsAg at week 12 and 24 of the treatment

Authors	HBeAg	HBsAg (IU/mL)	SVR Week		NPV Week	
			12	24	12	24
Chan et al,[32] 2010	Positive	<300	na[a]	62%	na[a]	na[a]
		>1 log decline	na[a]	75%	na[a]	85%
Lau et al,[34] 2009	Positive	>20,000	16%	15%	na[a]	na[a]
		<1500	57%	54%	72%	76%
Gane et al,[35] 2011	Positive	>20,000	0%	0%	84%	na[a]
		<1500	58%	57%	na[a]	na[a]
Sonneveld et al,[36] 2010	Positive	No decline	3%	8%	97%	na[a]
Piratvisuth et al,[37] 2011	Positive	No decline	18%	na[a]	82%	na[a]
Piratvisuth et al,[49] 2010	Positive	<1500	57%	na[a]		na[a]
Liaw et al,[50] 2011	Positive	<1500	57%	54%	84%	85%
		>20,000	0%	0%	100%	100%
Ma et al,[51] 2010	Positive	<1500	33%	na[a]	91%	na[a]
		<2890	na[a]	43%	na[a]	95%
Rijckborst et al,[43] 2010	Negative	Decline Yes[b]	39%	na[a]	na[a]	na[a]
		Decline No[b]	24%	na[a]	100%	na[a]
Moucari et al,[45] 2009	Negative	<0.5 log decline	88%	92%	90%	97%
Rijckborst et al,[52] 2012	Negative	No decline[b]	0%–5%	na[a]	95%–100%	na[a]
Lampertico et al,[53] 2011	Negative	≤7500	na[a]	17%	na[a]	na[a]
		>7500	na[a]	7%	na[a]	na[a]
Brunetto et al,[54] 2008	Negative	≥10 decline	47%	43%	na[a]	na[a]
		<10 decline	16%	13%	na[a]	na[a]

[a] Not available.
[b] Associated with < 2 log decrease in HBV DNA from baseline.

propose a response-guided therapy algorithm based on HBsAg kinetics at week 12 of treatment. Early identification of nonresponders would allow discontinuation of therapy and/or changing the treatment strategy (see **Table 1**).

NUCLEOS(T)IDES ANALOGUES

The goal of treatment with NAs is to maintain HBV suppression. Indeed, the newer agents such as tenofovir disoproxil fumarate (TDF) or entecavir (ETV) are more effective in suppressing HBV and are less likely to be associated with drug resistance than original NA. In addition, they are orally administered and have GOOD safety profile. However, they must probably be taken indefinitely because withdrawal is generally associated with viral reactivation, and HBsAg seroconversion is rarely reported. Although HBV DNA becomes rapidly undetectable, studies have clearly shown that the decline in HBsAg titers is significantly lower with NA therapy than with IFN-based treatment (**Fig. 4**).[57,58] Furthermore, the study of Boglione and colleagues[59] reports a significant difference in HBsAg levels decline at 2 years of therapy, according to the NAs administered (**Fig. 5**). Several studies have reported that baseline HBsAg levels and on treatment HBsAg quantification are good predictive markers of the end of treatment response and SVR.[57–67] Zoutendijk and colleagues[68] investigated HBsAg kinetics in patients who were successfully treated with long-term ETV or TDF. The authors used linear mixed regression analysis of individual HBsAg declines to estimate the duration of therapy required to achieve an HBsAg decline

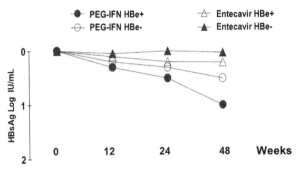

Fig. 4. Changes in HBsAg levels in HBeAg(+) and HBeAg(−) patients during PEG-IFN or ETV therapy. Mean changes compared with baseline for HBsAg titers in patients receiving either peginterferon or ETV therapy. The kinetics shows sharper decrease in patients receiving peginterferon therapy than in patients receiving ETV therapy independently from AgHBe status. Similar results are reported in HBeAg(−) chronic hepatitis B patients receiving either interferon or lamivudine.[58] (*Data from* Reijnders JG, Rijckborst V, Sonneveld MJ, et al. Kinetics of hepatits B surface antigen differ between treatment with peginterferon and entecavir. J Hepatol 2011;54:449–54.)

of 1 $\log_{10}$ UI/mL from baseline and HBsAg clearance. They showed that the median durations of therapy to achieve a 1 $\log_{10}$ IU/mL decrease were 6.6[1.7–18] years and 8[0.5–15] years in HBeAg(+) and HBeAg(−) patients, respectively. Median durations for HBsAg clearance were 36[10–93] years and 39[1.3–90] years in HBeAg(+) and HBeAg(−) patients, respectively. These results show the importance of determining HBsAg cutoffs to discontinue NA therapy with lowest risk of reactivation.

In the 2 pivotal studies of TDF, study in HBeAg(−)[69] and in HBeAg(+)[70] patients, the authors confirm that HBsAg kinetics is more deeper in HBeAg(+) patients than in HBeAg(−) and in patients receiving TDF monotherapy. The only patients with HBsAg loss were HBeAg(+) patients with a higher than 2 $\log_{10}$ IU/mL HBsAg decrease from baseline at 24 weeks of therapy, a higher baseline HBsAg level, and genotypes A or D. In a cohort of 162 HBeAg(+) patients with HBV DNA less than 60 IU/mL after 3 years of telbivudine therapy, Wursthorn and colleagues[63] showed that 25% of patients with greater than or equal to 1 $\log_{10}$ IU/mL HBsAg decrease after 1 year of therapy had an

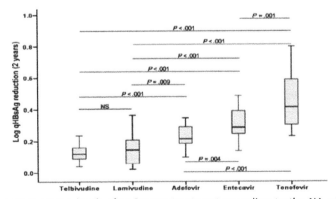

Fig. 5. Changes in HBsAg levels after 2 years treatment according to the NA administered. There are significant differences among qHBsAg kinetics from baseline to 2 years with different NAs. TDF showed the highest decline (0.45 log UI/mL), whereas ETV shows a moderate decline (0.38 log IU/mL), LdT (0.12 log IU/mL), ADV (0.22 log IU/mL), and LAM (0.14 log IU/mL).

HBsAg loss compared with 1.4% of patients with less than 1 $\log_{10}$ IU/mL HBsAg decrease. In a study by Reijnders and colleagues[58] in HBeAg(+) or HBeAg(−) patients, who received 48 weeks of either PEG-IFN or ETV, an HBsAg decline was only observed in HBeAg(+) patients after 48 weeks of either PEG-IFN or ETV therapy. In HBeAg(−) patients no decline in HBsAg levels was observed in patients receiving ETV. Recent studies including treatment-naive patients receiving NA report that low-baseline HBsAg levels and an early decline inHBsAg (24 weeks therapy) are good predictors of SVR.[64–67] Furthermore, studies suggest that an HBsAg cutoff lower than 2 to 3 $\log_{10}$ IU/mL could be used for treatment discontinuation.[71–74] In the study by Liang and colleagues,[71] 121 consecutive patients were prospectively recruited after treatment was stopped (lamivudine, ADV, ETV). The authors report that higher HBsAg levels at the end of treatment were associated with higher risk of relapse. End of treatment HBsAg levels less than or equal to 3 $\log_{10}$ IU/mL and less than or equal to 2 $\log_{10}$ IU/mL were associated with a 31% and 9% relapse, respectively. Similar results are reported by Cai and colleagues[74] in patients receiving 2 years of telbivudine therapy. An HBsAg level less than or equal to 2 IU/mL at the end of treatment cessation had a PPV and an NPV for the prediction of SVR of 100% and 93%, respectively.

ADD ON THERAPY

At least 2 studies report that the addition of PEG-IFN to ETV or TDF increases the on-treatment HBsAg decline, HBeAg seroconversion, and rate of SVR.[75,76]

HEPATITIS DELTA

The recent study of Wedemeyer and colleagues[77] showed that in hepatitis delta patients' treatment with the combination of PEG-IFN plus ADV was associated, more frequently, with an HBsAg decline higher than 1 log IU per milliliter at week 48 than in patients receiving mono therapy with ADV of PEG-IFN plus placebo (**Fig. 6**).

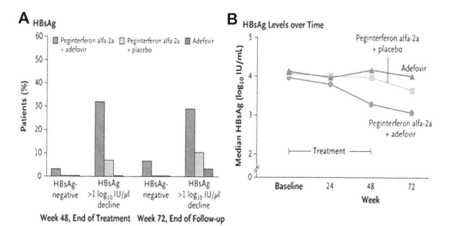

Fig. 6. Changes in HBsAg levels according to treatment in hepatitis delta patients. Patients received PEG-IFN plus ADV, PEG-IFN plus placebo, or ADV alone. (*A*) Percentage of patients, in each treatment group, with an HBsAg decline higher than 1 log IU/mL or HBsAg clearance achieved at week 48 or week 72. (*B*) Decline of HBsAg according to treatment. Decline was significantly steeper in patients receiving the combination therapy than in patients receiving PEG-IFN plus placebo or ADV mono-therapy (P = .002 at week 248 and P<. 001 at week 72).

SUMMARY

Several recent studies on serum HBsAg monitoring show that HBsAg levels change during the natural course of CHB and during ongoing therapy. These results can be used to determine the best management strategy for patients. During the natural history of HBV, HBsAg quantification can be used to differentiate between inactive carriers (no need for treatment) and HBeAg(−) CHB patients, who are likely to reactivate (closer monitoring) and who can benefit from therapy. During PEG-IFN therapy early HBsAg monitoring could be used to develop a response-guided algorithm to stop or switch therapy at week 12 in poor responders, to continue standard 48-week treatment in most patients with a favorable response, and to extend therapy for intermediate on-treatment responders to improve the chances of response. The role of HBsAg monitoring during NA therapy must be clarified. The development of stopping rules should be determined in these lifelong therapies. Several studies suggest that baseline treatment and on-treatment HBsAg levels might help identify patients who can stop therapy with reduced risk of reactivation.

REFERENCES

1. Ganem D, Prince AM. Hepatitis B virus infection-natural history and clinical consequences. N Engl J Med 2004;350:118–29.
2. McMahon BJ. The natural history of chronic hepatitis B virus infection. Hepatology 2009;49:S45–55.
3. Werle-Lapostolle B, Bowden S, Locarnini S, et al. Persistence of cccDNA during the natural history of chronic hepatitis B and decline during adefovir dipivoxil therapy. Gastroenterology 2004;126:1750–8.
4. Madalinski K, Burczynska B, Heermann KH, et al. Analysis of viral proteins in circulating immune complexes from chronic carriers of hepatitis B virus. Clin Exp Immunol 1991;84:493–500.
5. Chan HL, Wong VW, Tse AM, et al. Serum hepatitis B surface antigen quantitation can reflect hepatitis B virus in the liver and predict treatment response. Clin Gastroenterol Hepatol 2007;5:1462–8.
6. Nguyen T, Thompson AJ, Bowden S, et al. Hepatitis B surface antigen levels during the natural history of chronic hepatitis B: a perspective on Asia. J Hepatol 2010;52:508–13.
7. Thompson AJ, Nguyen T, Iser D, et al. Serum hepatitis B surface antigen and hepatitis B e antigen titers: disease phase influences correlation with viral load and intrahepatic hepatitis B virus markers. Hepatology 2010;51:1933–44.
8. Jaroszewicz J, Calle Serrano B, Wursthorn K, et al. Hepatitis B surface antigen (HBsAg) levels in the natural history of hepatitis B virus (HBV)-infection: a European perspective. J Hepatol 2010;52:514–22.
9. Wursthorn K, Jaroszewicz J, Zacher BJ, et al. Correlation between the Elecsys HBsAg II assay and the architect assay for quantification of hepatitis B surface antigen (HBsAg) in serum. J Clin Virol 2011;50:292–6.
10. Sonneveld MJ, Rijckborst V, Boucher CA, et al. A comparison of two assays for quantification of hepatitis B surface antigen in patients with chronic hepatitis B. J Clin Virol 2011;51:175–8.
11. Liaw YF. Clinical utility of hepatitis B surface antigen quantification in patients with chronic hepatitis B: a review. Hepatology 2011;53:2121–9.
12. Chan HL, Wong GL, Wong VW. A review of the natural history of chronic hepatitis B in the era of transient elastography. Antivir Ther 2009;14:489–99.

13. Martinot-Peignoux M, Lapalus M, Lada O, et al. Natural history of hepatitis B (HBV) infection: role of HBV genotype (A to E) assessed in a large cohort. Hepatology 2011;54(Suppl):609A.
14. Chan HL, Thompson A, Martinot-Peignoux, et al. Hepatitis B surface antigen quantification: why and how to use it in 2011-A core group report. J Hepatol 2011;55:1121–31.
15. Brunetto MR, Oliveri F, Rocca G, et al. Natural course and response to interferon of chronic hepatitis B accompaned by antibody to hepatitis B e antigen. Hepatology 1989;10:198–202.
16. Sung JJ, Chan HL, Wong ML, et al. Relationship of clinical and virological factors with hepatitis activity in hepatitis B e antigen-negative chronic hepatitis B virus-infected patients. J Viral Hepat 2002;9:229–34.
17. Martinot-Peignoux M, Boyer N, Colombat M, et al. Serum hepatitis B virus HBV DNA levels and liver histology in inactive HBsAg carriers. J Hepatol 2002;36:543–6.
18. Brunetto MR, Oiveri F, Coco B, et al. Outcome of anti-HBe positive chronic hepatitis B in alpha-interferon and untreated patients: a long term cohort study. J Hepatol 2002;36:263–70.
19. Papatheodoridis GV, Manesis EK, Manalakopoulos S, et al. Is there a meaninful serum hepatitis B virus DNA cutoff level for therapeutic decisions in hepatitis B e antigen-negative chronic hepatitis B infection? Hepatology 2008;48:1451–9.
20. Lok AS, Heathcote EJ, Hoofnagle JH. Management of hepatitis B: 2000-summary of a workshop. Gastroenterology 2001;120:1828–53.
21. European Association for the Study of the Liver. EASL clinical practice guidelines: management of chronic hepatitis B. J Hepatol 2012;50:227–42.
22. Chan HL, Wong VW, Wong GL, et al. A longitudinal study on the natural history of serum HBsAg changes in chronic hepatitis B. Hepatology 2010;52:1232–41.
23. Chan HL, Wong GL, Tse CH, et al. Definition of inactive hepatitis B carrer by serum HBsAg and HBV DNA levels - a long-term follow-up study on HBsAg seroclearance. J Hepatol 2011;54:S144.
24. Brunetto MR, Oliveri F, Colombatto P, et al. Hepatitis B surface antigen serum levels help to distinguish active from inactive hepatitis B virus genotype D carriers. Gastroenterology 2010;139:483–90.
25. Martinot-Peignoux M, Lada O, Cardoso AC, et al. Quantitative HBsAg: a new specific marker for the diagnosis of HBsAg inactive carriage. Hepatology 2010;52:992A.
26. Martinot-Peignoux M, Lapalus M, Laouénan C, et al. How to distinguish HBeAg negative chronic hepatitis B, with high risk of reactivation, from inactive carriers: is there a place for HBsAg quantification? Hepatology 2012;56(Suppl):434A.
27. Seto WK, Wnog DK, Fung J, et al. High hepatitis B surface antigen levels predict insignificant fibrosis in hepatitis B e antigen positive chronic hepatitis B. PLoS One 2012;7:e43087.
28. Martinot-Peignoux M, Carvalho RJ, Cardoso AC, et al. Hepatitis B surface antigen serum level is associated with fibrosis severity in treatment-naive, e-antigen-positive patients. J Hepatol 2013;58(6):1089–95.
29. Lau GK, Piratvisuth T, Luo KX, et al. Peginterferon alfa-2a, lamuvidine, and the combination for HbeAg-positive chronic hepatitis B. N Engl J Med 2005;352:2682–95.

30. Marcellin P, Lau GK, Bonino F, et al. Peginterferon alfa-2a, lamuvidine, and the two in combination for HBeAg-negative chronic hepatitis B. N Engl J Med 2004; 351:1206–17.

31. Janssen HL, Kerhof-Los CJ, Heijtink RA, et al. Measurement of HBsAg to monitor hepatitis B viral replication in patients on α-interferon therapy. Antiviral Res 1994;23:251–7.

32. Chan HL, Wong VW, Chim AM, et al. Serum HBsAg quantification to predict response to peginterferon therapy of e antigen positive chronic hepatitis B. Aliment Pharmacol Ther 2010;32:1323–31.

33. Tangkijvanich P, Komolmit P, Mahachai V, et al. Low pretreatment serum HBsAg level and viral mutations as predictors of response to Peginterferon alfa-2b therapy in chronic hepatitis B. J Clin Virol 2009;46:117–23.

34. Lau G, Marcellin P, Brunetto M. On treatment monitoring of HBsAg levels to predict response to peginterferon alfa-2a in patients with HBeAg-positive Chronic hepatitis B. J Hepatol 2009;50:S333.

35. Gane E, Jia J, Han K, et al. NEPTUNE study; on treatment HBs Ag level analysis confirms prediction of response observed in phase 3 study of peginterferon alfa-2a in HBeAg positive patients. J Hepatol 2011;54:Abstract 69.

36. Sonneveld MJ, Rijckborst V, Boucher CA, et al. Prediction of sustained response to peginterferon alfa-2b for hepatitis B e antigen-positive chronic hepatitis B using on-treatment hepatitis B surface antigen decline. Hepatology 2010;52:1251–7.

37. Piratvisuth T, Marcellin P. Further analysis is required to identify an early stopping rule for peginterferon therapy that is valid for all HBeAg-positive patients. Hepatology 2011;53:1054–5.

38. Flink HJ, van Zonneveld M, Hansen B, et al. treatment with Peg-Interferon a-2a for HBeAg-positive chronic hepatitis B: HBsAg loss is associated with HBV genotype? Am J Gastroenterol 2006;101:297–303.

39. Soneveld MJ, Rijckborst V, Cakalog-1 lu Y, et al. Durable hepatitis surface antigen decline in hepatitis B e antigen positive chronic hepatitis B patients treated with pegylated interferon-a2b: relation to response and HBV genotype. Antivir Ther 2012;17:9–17.

40. Moucari R, Martinot-Peignoux M, Mackiewicz V, et al. Influence of genotype on hepatitis B surafce antigen in hepatitis B e antigen-negative patients trated with pegylated interferon-a2a. Antivir Ther 2009;14:1183–8.

41. Hadziyannis SJ. Treatment paradigms on hepatitis Be antigen-negative chronic hepatitis B patients. Expert Opin Investig Drugs 2007;16:777–86.

42. Bonino F, Marcellin P, Lau GK, et al. Predicting response to peginterferon alpha-2a, lamivudine and the two combined for HBeAg-negative chronic hepatitis B. Gut 2007;56:699–705.

43. Rijckborst V, Hansen BE, Cakalog-1 lu Y, et al. Early on-treatment prediction of response to peginterferon alfa-2a for HBeAg-negative chronic hepatitis B using HBsAg and HBV DNA levels. Hepatology 2010;52:454–61.

44. Marcellin P, Bonino F, Lau GK, et al. Sustained response of hepatitis B e antigen-negative patients 3 years after treatment with peginterferon alpha-2a. Gastroenterology 2009;136:2169–79.

45. Moucari R, Mackiewicz V, Lada O, et al. Early serum HBsAg drop: a strong predictor of sustained virological response to pegylated interferon alfa-2a in HBeAg-negative patients. Hepatology 2009;49:1151–7.

46. Brunetto MR, Moriconi F, Bononi F, et al. Hepatitis B virus surface antigen levels: a guide to sutained response to peginterferon alfa-2a in HBeAg-negative chronic hepatitis B. Hepatology 2009;49:1141–50.

47. Moucari R. Peginterferon for chronic hepatitis B: predicting success with on-treatment benchmarks. J Gastroenterol Hepatol 2010;25:1474–5.
48. Moucari R, Korevaar A, Lada O, et al. High rates of HBsAg seroconversion in HBeAg-positive chronic hepatitis B patients responding to interferon: a long-term follow-up study. J Hepatol 2009;50:1084–92.
49. Piratvisuth T, Lau GK, Marvellin P, et al. On-treatment decline in serum HBsAg levels predicts sustained immune control and HBsAg clearance 6 month post-treatment in HBsAg positive hepatitisB virus-infected patients treated with peginterferon alfa-2a (40kD) (PEGASYS). Hepatol Int 2010;4:152.
50. Liaw YF, Jia JD, Chan HL, et al. Shorter duration and lower doses of peginterferon alfa-2a are associated with inferior hepatitis Be antigen seroconversion rates in hepatitis B virus genotypes B or C. Hepatology 2011;54:1591–9.
51. Ma H, Yang RF, Wei L. Quantitative serum HBsAg and HBaAg are strong predictors of sustained HBeAg seroconversion to pegylated interferon alfa 2b in HbeAg positive patients. J Gard Hist 2010;25:1498–506.
52. Rijckborst V, Hansen BE, Ferenci P, et al. Validation of a stopping rule at week 12 using HBsAg and HBV DNA for HBeAg-negative patients treated with peginterferon alpha-2a. J Hepatol 2012;6:1006–11.
53. Lampertico P, Vigano M, Di Costanzo GC, et al. Response-guided peginterferon alfa-2a therapy based on HBsAg levels at week 12 and week 24 or 48 improves respose rates in HBeAg negative genotype D patients. J Hepatol 2011;56:S207.
54. Brunetto M, Bonino F, Marcellin P, et al. Kinetics of HBsAg decline in patients with HBeAg negative chronic hepatitis B treated with peginterferon alfa 2a according to genotype and its association woth sustained HBsAg clearance. Hepatology 2008;48(Suppl):740A.
55. Lampertico P, Liaw YF. New perspectives in the therapy of chronic hepatitis B. Gut 2012;61(Suppl 1):i18–24.
56. Lampertico P, Vigano P, Di Costanzo G, et al. Extended (2 years) treatment with peginterferon alfa-2a improves sustained response rates in genotype D patients with HBeAg negative chronic hepatitis B. J Hepatol 2010;52:S45.
57. Manesis EK, Hadziyannis ES, Angelopoulou OS, et al. Prediction of treatment-related HBsAg loss in HBeAg-negative chronic hepatitis B: a clue from serum HBsAg levels. Antivir Ther 2007;12:73–82.
58. Reijnders JG, Rijckborst V, Sonneveld MJ, et al. Kinetics of hepatits B surface antigen differ between treatment with peginterferon and entecavir. J Hepatol 2011;54:449–54.
59. Boglione L, D'Avolio A, Cariti G, et al. Kinetics and prediction of HBsAg loss during therapy with analogues i patients affected by chronic hepatitis B HBeAg negative and genotype D. Liver Int 2013;33(4):580–5.
60. Lee MH, Lee DM, Kim SS, et al. Correlation of serum hepatitis B srface antigen level with response to entecavir in naive patients with chronic hepatitis B. J Med Virol 2011;83:1178–86.
61. Lee JM, Ahn SH, Kim HS, et al. Quantitative hepatitis B surface antigen and hepatitis B e atigen titers in prediction of treatment response to entecavir. Hepatology 2011;53:1486–93.
62. Chen J, Wang Z, Zhou B, et al. Factors associated with hepatitis B surface antigen levels and its on-treatment changes in patients under lamivudine therapy. Antivir Ther 2012;17:71–9.
63. Wursthorn K, Jung M, Riva A, et al. Kinetics of hepatitis B surface antigen decline during 3 years of telbivudine treatment in hepatitis B e antigen-positive patients. Hepatology 2010;52:1611–20.

64. Gramenzi A, Log-1 gi E, Micco L, et al. Serum hepatitis B surface antigen monitiring in long-term lamuvudine-treated hepatitis B virus patients. J Viral Hepat 2011;10:468–74.

65. Zoulim F, Carosi G, Greenbloom S, et al. Quantification of HBsAg in nucleos(t)ides-naive patients treated for chronic hepatitis B with entecavir or entecavir plus tenofovir in the BE-LOW study. J Viral Hepat 2012; 19(Suppl S3):O224.

66. Bruce MJ, Horner M, Knighton S, et al. Strong decline in HBsAg levels after virological response in a large monocentric therapy cohort: potential to select HBeAg positive chronic hepatitis B patients for finite duration? Hepatology 2012;56(Suppl):439A.

67. Orito E, Kusakabe A, Kanie H, et al. Quantification of HBsAg predicts response to naive entrcavir therapy in chronic hepatitis B patients with genotype C. Hepatology 2012;56(Suppl):395A.

68. Zoutendijk R, Hansen BE, Van Vuuren AJ, et al. Prediction of HBsAg loss using HBsAg decline after long-term virological response to nucleos(t)ide analogue therapy for chronic hepatitis B. Hepatology 2010;52:Abstract 38.

69. Marcellin M, Heathcote EJ, Buti M, et al. Tenofovir Disiproxil Fumarate versus adefovir dipivoxil for chronic hepatitis B. N Engl J Med 2008;359:2442–55.

70. Heathcote EJ, Marcellin M, Buti M, et al. Three years efficacy and safety of Tenofovir Disiproxil Fumarate treatment for chronic hepatitis B. Gastroenterology 2011;140:132–43.

71. Liang Y, Jiang J, Su M, et al. Predictors of relapse in chronic hepatitis B after discontinuation of antiviral therapy. Aliment Pharmacol Ther 2011;34:344–52.

72. Petersen J, Buggischi P, Stoehr A, et al. Stopping long-term nucleos(t)ides analogue therapy before HBsAg loss or seroconversion in HBeAg negative CHB patients: experience from five referral centers in Germany. Hepatology 2011;54(Suppl):1417A.

73. Suh SJ, Yeon JE, Yoon EL, et al. Quantification of serum hepatitis B surface antigen as a predictor of off-treatment sustained virological response in in chronic hepatitis B patients treated with oral nucleos(t)ide analogue. J Hepatol 2012;56: S191.

74. Cai W, Xie Q, An B, et al. On-treatment serum HBsAg level is predictive of sustained off-treatment virologic response to telbivudine in HBeAg-positive chronic hepatitis B patients. J Clin Virol 2010;48:22–6.

75. Marcellin P, Martinot-Peignoux M, Lapalus M, et al. Week 12 HBsAg titer decline is predictive of SVR in chronic hepatitis B patients receiving pegylated inteferon plus teneofovir combination therapy. J Hepatol 2012;56:S71–224.

76. Sooneveld ML, Qing X, Zhang NP, et al. Adding peginterferon alfa-2a to entecavir increases HBsAd decline and HBsAg clearance-first results from a global randomized trial. Hepatology 2012;4(Suppl):199A.

77. Wedemeyer H, Yurdayin C, Dalekos GN, et al. Peginterferon plus adefovir versus either drug alone for hepatitis delta. N Engl J Med 2011;364:322–31.

Impact of Therapy on the Long-Term Outcome of Chronic Hepatitis B

Yun-Fan Liaw, MD

KEYWORDS

- Cirrhosis • Hepatic decompensation • Hepatic fibrosis • Hepatocellular carcinoma
- Interferon • Nucleos(t)ide analog

KEY POINTS

- The ultimate goal of chronic hepatitis B therapy is to reduce disease progression and prolong life.
- Both interferon-based finite therapy and long-term Nuc therapy may improve hepatic fibrosis, reduce disease progression including HCC development, and prolong survival.
- Sustained or maintained response and viral suppression are crucial for better long-term outcomes. Therefore, entecavir and tenofovir disoproxil fumarate are preferred Nucs because of the low risk of drug resistance.
- Pegylated interferon therapy increases hepatitis B surface antigen seroclearance over time to reach a status closest to a cure.

INTRODUCTION

Chronic hepatitis B virus (HBV) infection is a dynamic state of interactions between HBV, the hepatocytes, and the immune system of the host. Patients with an extended immune clearance phase may develop adverse sequelae such as hepatic decompensation and cirrhosis or hepatocellular carcinoma (HCC).[1] Studies have shown that active HBV replication is the key driving force for the subsequent HBV-related immune clearance events that determine the clinical outcome.[1,2] Therefore, the primary aim of therapy is to eliminate or permanently suppress HBV to reduce hepatitis activity and thereby reduce the risk or slow the progression of liver disease. The ultimate long-term goal is to achieve a sustained response to prevent or reduce the development of hepatic decompensation, cirrhosis, or HCC and prolong survival,[3–5] as summarized in **Fig. 1**. The advent of effective antiviral agents with different mechanisms of action

Disclosure: YF Liaw has been involved with clinical trials and served as a global advisory board member of Roche, BMS, Novartis, Gilead Sciences.
Liver Research Unit, Chang Gung Memorial Hospital, Chang Gung University College of Medicine, 199, Tung Hwa North Road, Taipei 105, Taiwan
E-mail address: liveryfl@gmail.com

Clin Liver Dis 17 (2013) 413–423
http://dx.doi.org/10.1016/j.cld.2013.05.005　　　　　　　　　　**liver.theclinics.com**
1089-3261/13/$ – see front matter © 2013 Elsevier Inc. All rights reserved.

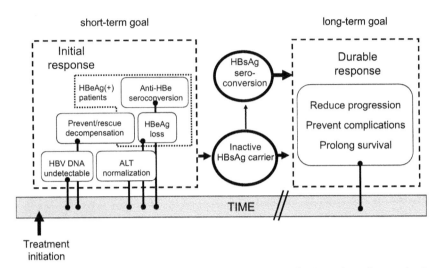

short-term goal

long-term goal

Fig. 1. Goals of treatment of patients with chronic HBV infection. The primary aim is to permanently suppress HBV replication to achieve biochemical, serologic, and histologic improvement, to prevent or rescue hepatic decompensation and ultimately reduce progression of liver disease, prevent complications, and prolong survival. (*Adapted from* Liaw YF, Kao JH, Piratvisuth T, et al. Asian-Pacific consensus statement on the management of chronic hepatitis B: a 2012 update. Hepatol Int 2012;6:531–61; with permission.)

has provided opportunities to achieve these goals. Evidence has shown that anti-HBV therapy may improve the long-term outcomes of chronic HBV infection.

ANTIVIRAL THERAPY FOR CHRONIC HBV INFECTION

Currently, conventional interferon α (IFN), pegylated interferon α_{2a} (Peg IFN), lamivudine (LAM), adefovir dipivoxil (ADV), entecavir (ETV), telbivudine, and tenofovir disoproxil fumarate (TDF) have been approved for the treatment of chronic HBV infection. Short-term studies have shown that IFN-based therapy is modestly efficacious in inducing hepatitis B e antigen (HBeAg) loss or seroconversion (30–40%) in patients with HBeAg-positive chronic hepatitis B (CHB)[6,7] and in producing sustained HBV DNA suppression (<20,000 copies/mL) in ~40% of HBeAg-negative patients.[8–11] Therapy with direct antiviral nucleos(t)ide analog (Nuc) may suppress HBV replication rapidly and profoundly in both HBeAg-positive and HBeAg-negative patients followed by normalization of serum alanine aminotransferase (ALT) levels and significant improvement in liver disease, including reversion of fibrosis.[12–16] A critical review of 26 therapeutic trials involving 3428 patients showed that treatment-induced HBV DNA reduction correlated significantly and consistently with histologic, biochemical, and serologic responses, especially in studies using direct antiviral agents and in HBeAg-positive patients.[17]

IMPACT OF ANTI-HBV THERAPY ON LONG-TERM OUTCOMES
IFN-Based Therapy

HBeAg-positive CHB
Long-term follow-up studies after a 4- to 6-month course of IFN therapy in HBeAg-positive patients showed reduction in fibrosis progression, especially in sustained

HBeAg seroconverters. A large study comparing 233 IFN-treated HBeAg-positive patients with 233 well-matched (for age, sex, ALT, HBeAg status, histology, and length of follow-up) untreated patients did show a reduced cumulative incidence of cirrhosis (17.8% vs 33.7% in the controls; P = .041) during a median follow-up period of 6.8 years (range 1.1–15.5 years).[18] Studies also showed that sustained elimination of HBeAg was associated with a significant increase in survival[6,18,19] and a reduction in the occurrence of severe cirrhotic complications and the need for liver transplantation.[19] More data, including an earlier randomized control study,[6] showed that IFN therapy in HBeAg-positive active chronic hepatitis reduced the incidence (2.7% vs 12.5% in controls during 1.1 to 15.5 years follow-up; P = .011) of HCC development.[18]

HBeAg-negative CHB
In HBeAg-negative European patients treated with IFN for 6 to 24 months, sustained responders also showed decreased progression of Ishak fibrosis score[8,9] or decreased risk of cirrhosis.[20] Sustained responders also had significantly improved long-term outcomes, including less severe cirrhosis-related complications, reduced incidence of HCC (1.8% vs 10.5% in relapsers; P = .027% and 7.7% in untreated; P = .048), less need for liver transplantation, and lower mortality, although the sustained response rate in HBeAg-negative patients was usually lower than 30%.[8,9,20] In a 3-year follow-up study after the end of Peg IFN therapy in HBeAg-negative patients, only 1 of 230 patients (55 with Metavir fibrosis score 3 or 4) developed HCC.[11]

CHB with cirrhosis
It has been shown that IFN-based therapy in compensated cirrhotic patients is safe and even more effective than in noncirrhotic patients.[21,22] This finding suggests that the benefit of reducing HCC in cirrhotic patients might be evident with longer follow-up after IFN-based therapy. A subgroup analysis in a long-term follow-up study did show that HCC incidence was reduced significantly in IFN-treated cirrhotic patients.[18] A meta-analysis involving 12 trials (1292 patients treated with IFN and 1450 untreated) showed that the risk of HCC was significantly reduced by 34% (relative risk [RR] 0.66, 95% confidence interval [CI] 0.48–0.89; P = .006) after treatment with IFN, and even higher (47% reduction; RR 0.53, 95% CI 0.36–0.78; P = .001) in cirrhotic patients.[23] Another meta-analysis involving 11 trials also showed that IFN therapy had a beneficial effect in reducing cirrhosis (RR 0.65; 95% CI 0.47–0.91; P = .01) and HCC (RR 0.59; 95% CI 0.43–0.81; P = .001).[24] The pooled estimated of another meta-analysis involving 2 randomized control trials (RCTs) and 5 non-randomized controlled trials (553 treated with IFN vs 750 with no treatment) showed a significant preventive effect on HCC development in favor of IFN therapy, especially in HBeAg-positive patients, Asian patients, or in a population with higher HCC incidence.[25] With the beneficial long-term effect of IFN-based therapy in reducing cirrhosis and HCC development, cirrhotic complications or HCC and liver death are also reduced (RR 0.55; 95% CI 0.43–0.70; P<.001).[26]

Direct Antiviral Therapy

Impact on hepatic fibrosis
Long-term (>3 years) LAM or ADV therapy resulted in improvement of fibrosis or reversal of advanced fibrosis.[12,13,27] There was a significantly lower cumulative rate of cirrhosis and/or development of HCC (P = .005) with long-term LAM therapy (median 89.9 months; range 26.5–128.3 months) in 142 HBeAg-positive noncirrhotic patients from Hong Kong compared with 124 HBeAg-positive untreated controls.[28] With a low incidence of drug resistance, long-term therapy with ETV or TDF results

in maintained undetectable serum HBV DNA in more than 90% of patients.[16,29] Fibrosis improved ($\geq$1 point on the Ishak fibrosis score) in 57% and 88% of patients treated with ETV for 3 and 6 years, respectively.[30,31] Significant regression of fibrosis or cirrhosis was also observed in 51% of 348 patients (74% of 96 patients with cirrhosis at baseline) treated with TDF for 5 years.[16] **Table 1** summarizes the data on fibrosis regression during various Nuc therapies.

Impact on liver disease progression, decompensation, and survival

A double-blind RCT showed that maintenance LAM therapy for a median of 32.4 months in 436 patients with advanced fibrosis or cirrhosis (Ishak fibrosis score $\geq$4) significantly reduced overall disease progression (17.7% vs 7.8%; $P = .001$) compared with 215 untreated controls.[32] Long-term therapy with a Nuc with a low genetic barrier such as LAM was associated with a high rate of drug-resistant mutations.[3–5] Patients with drug resistance were more likely to experience disease progression and die from causes related to the worsening of liver function, especially in patients with advanced fibrosis or cirrhosis.[32] This adverse outcome can be rescued now. The 5-year cumulative incidence of hepatic decompensation in Korean patients with compensated cirrhosis reduced from 45.4% in 481 untreated historical control patients to 15.4% in 150 patients who were treated with LAM and rescue therapy when needed ($P<.001$). The 5-year cumulative survival of the treated patients was 90.9% in contrast to 74.3% ($P = .001$) of the untreated controls.[33] None of the 94 cirrhotic patients from Italy treated with LAM and rescued with ADV developed hepatic decompensation for up to 4 years.[34] For a Nuc with very low drug resistance, a multicenter study in Italy showed that none of the Nuc-naive patients with compensated cirrhosis treated with ETV for 53 months (range 2–74 months) died of hepatic decompensation.[35] The VIRGIL study also showed that virological response (serum HBV DNA <80 IU/mL) to ETV therapy during a median duration of 20 months (range 11–32 months) was associated with a 71% reduction in the probability of developing decompensations, HCC, or death when compared with those who failed to maintain a virological response.[36] For patients with decompensated cirrhosis in Korea, Nuc therapy starting with LAM resulted in a significantly higher 5-year cumulative survival in Child B (62.8 vs 33.5% in controls; $P = .003$) and Child C (62.2% vs 10.2% in controls; $P<.001$) patients with cirrhosis.[33]

Impact on HCC development

Patients with advanced fibrosis or cirrhosis are more prone to develop clinical end points such as HCC. Thus, it is easier and requires shorter duration to demonstrate

Table 1
Fibrosis regression during long-term therapy with nucleos(t)ide analogs

Nucleos(t)ide	No.	HBeAg	Duration (y)	Fibrosis Regression (%)	Reference
Lamivudine	63	+	3	33	[12]
Entecavir	21	+ or −	3	57	[30]
Adefovir	24	−	5	71	[13]
Adefovir	15	+	5	60	[27]
Entecavir	57	+ or −	6[a]	88	[31]
Tenofovir	348/96[b]	+ or −	5	51/74[b]	[16]

[a] Median time of long-term biopsy: 6 years (range 3–7 years).
[b] Patients with Ishak fibrosis score 5 and 6 at baseline.

the impact of Nuc therapy on HCC development in this patient population. In the RCT mentioned earlier, the incidence of HCC was also significantly reduced in the LAM-treated patients with advanced fibrosis or cirrhosis (3.9% vs 7.4% in the placebo group, $P = .048$).[32] A retrospective multicenter study involving 303 HBeAg-negative patients with liver cirrhosis treated with LAM for 1 to 66 months (median 22 months) showed that HBV suppression reduced the development of HCC, but the chance of developing HCC was significantly greater ($P<.001$) in patients with a virological break-through than in those who maintained viral suppression.[37] An earlier meta-analysis involving 1267 LAM-treated and 1022 untreated patients showed that HCC was reduced by 78% (RR 0.22, 95% CI 0.10–0.50; $P = .0003$) when LAM therapy was maintained and a greater benefit was observed in patients with cirrhosis and HBeAg-positive patients.[23] In a systemic review of 21 studies (starting with LAM in 19 studies) in 3881 Nuc-treated and 534 untreated patients, HCC developed less frequently in Nuc-treated patients (2.8% vs 6.4%; $P<.003$) and the benefit was greater in those with virological remission (2.3% vs 7.5%; $P<.001$) but the HCC incidence in Nuc-treated cirrhotic patients remained at 10.8% during a 46-month period.[38] More recent Asian studies also showed a reduced incidence of HCC in patients with compensated cirrhosis who achieved sustained viral suppression under LAM therapy, compared with untreated patients or LAM-treated patients with a viral breakthrough or a suboptimal response.[33,39,40] Since rescue therapy and Nucs with a high genetic barrier to drug resistance became available, the incidence of HCC has been reduced further. A study from Italy involving 94 patients treated with LAM and rescued with ADV when needed showed a 4-year cumulative incidence of HCC of 15% during a mean duration of 42 months on Nuc therapy.[34] A multicenter study from Greece on long-term (median 4.7 years) Nuc therapy starting with LAM showed a 5-year cumulative incidence of HCC of 9.2% and 19.3% in 160 HBeAg-negative patients with compen-sated cirrhosis and 56 with decompensated cirrhosis, respectively.[41] For ETV therapy, only 1 of 144 patients treated up to 5 years developed HCC at week 51 of treatment,[15] and only 3 of 372 patients (47% HBeAg positive, 98 cirrhotics) developed HCC during a median treatment period of 20 months in the VIRGIL study.[36] A large study from Japan has clearly shown that the 5-year cumulative incidence of HCC in cirrhotic pa-tients (43% HBeAg-positive) is much lower in ETV-treated patients compared with propensity score matched untreated controls and LAM-treated controls (7% vs 20% in LAM; $P = .043%$ and 38% in untreated controls; $P<.001$).[42] In 382 HBeAg-negative cirrhotic patients from Taiwan treated with ETV, the cumulative incidence of HCC was 7.3% during a mean follow-up of 35.9 months.[43] A multicenter study in Italy showed a 5-year cumulative incidence of HCC of 14% in 164 cirrhotic patients treated with ETV for 52 months (range 2–74 months).[34] The incidence of HCC in 152 patients with cirrhosis and 482 patients with CHB treated with TDF for 5 years was only 3.3% and 1.5%, respectively.[44] The beneficial impact of Nuc therapy on the development of HCC in cirrhotic patients is clearly demonstrated in studies with con-trol group(s), all from Asia where patients were mainly infected with genotype C or B HBV.[32,33,42] Better virological suppression also tends to reduce the annual incidence of HCC in European cohort studies in which the patients were mainly infected with ge-notype D.[34,35,37,41] In addition to the potency and genetic barrier to resistance of the Nuc used for therapy, different proportions of male gender, age, HBeAg serostatus, and HBV genotype of the patients included in different studies may also contribute to the different results shown in **Table 2** and **Fig. 2**. The importance of the age factor was clearly demonstrated in a study showing that the incidence of HCC during Nuc therapy was significantly higher in patients over 60 years than in those between 50 and 60 years of age than in those younger than 50 years of age.[41]

Table 2
HCC incidence in cirrhotic patients with HBV on anti-HBV therapy

Source	Study	Treatment	No.	Age (y)	Male (%)	HBeAg (-) (%)	Follow-Up	HCC (%)/No. of Years[a]
Liaw et al,[32] 2004	RCT	LAM	436 vs 215[b,c]	43 vs 44[b]	85	58	32.4 (0–42) mo	5 vs 10/3
Di Marco et al,[37] 2004	Cohort	LAM	303	52	88	100	22 (1–66) mo	19.8/3
Lampertico et al,[34] 2007	Cohort	LAM±R	94	58	84	86	42 (12–74) mo	15/4
Papatheodoridis et al,[41] 2011	Cohort	LAM±R	160	59	78	100	4.5 (3.7–5.0) y	9.2/5
Kurokawa et al,[40] 2012	Cohort	LAM±R	88	52	76	52	65.5 ± 29.5 mo	30/5
Kim et al,[33] 2012	HC	LAM±R	240 vs 481[b]	50 vs 46[b]	68	40	46.4 (1–124) mo	13.5 vs 23.4/5
Hosaka et al,[42] 2012	PSM	ETV vs LAM vs control	78 vs 49 vs 85[b]	46 vs 45 vs 46[b]	66 vs 75	57	3.3 (2.3–4.3) vs 6.8 (5–9.9) vs 7.6 (3.4–13.7) y	7.0 vs 22.2 vs 38.9/5
Lampertico et al,[35] 2012	Cohort	ETV	164	58	76	83	53 (2–74) mo	14/5
Chen et al,[43] 2013	Cohort	ETV	386	55	85	100	35.6 ± 1.39 mo	7.3/3
Buti et al,[44] 2012	Cohort	TDF	152	68% >40	81	38	~5 y (76%)	3.3/5
Marcellin et al,[11] 2009	Cohort	Peg IFN	55[d]	40	83	100	3 y	1.8/3

Abbreviations: ±R, with rescue therapy when indicated; HC, historical control; PSM, propensity score matched controls.
[a] Cumulative incidence for the number of years indicated.
[b] Data for untreated control patients.
[c] 260 versus 139 patients were cirrhotic; the remaining patients had Ishak fibrosis score 4.
[d] Patients with Metavir fibrosis score 3 and 4.

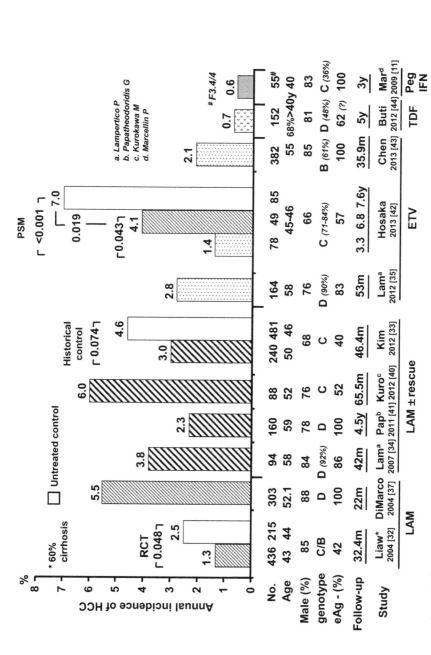

Fig. 2. The reported or calculated annual incidence of HCC in patients with hepatitis B and cirrhosis on long-term therapy with nucleos(t)ide analogs is lower than untreated controls. ETV is superior to LAM in reducing the development of HCC. PSM, propensity score matched control.

Overall conclusion on long-term impact

These results confirm that suppression of HBV reduces the risk or slows the progression of liver disease, and that renewed HBV replication may restore the potential for disease progression if not properly rescued. It is important to start therapy using a Nuc with a high genetic barrier, such as ETV or TDF, as the preferred first-line drug.[3–5]

Hepatitis B Surface Antigen Seroclearance as an Ideal Outcome

Hepatitis B surface antigen (HBsAg) seroclearance is a state closest to a cure of chronic HBV infection[45] and, therefore, is the ideal outcome of antiviral therapy. Long-term follow-up studies have shown that IFN-based therapy increases HBsAg seroclearance over time. HBsAg seroclearance occurred more frequently in patients with sustained response to IFN-based therapy[8–11,21] and was associated with a lower rate of hepatic decompensation and HCC, and with longer survival.[10] A 3-year (mean) follow-up study in 172 HBeAg-positive patients treated with Peg IFNα_{2b} showed that HBsAg seroclearance was achieved in 11% and 30% of patients overall and initial responders, respectively.[46] In 230 HBeAg-negative patients, the HBsAg seroclearance rate increased from 5% at 1 year to 9% at 3 years[11] and to 12% at 5 years (28% among initial responders) after Peg IFN α_{2a} therapy.[47] However, the HBsAg seroclearance rate was much lower (2.4%) in Asian patients treated with Peg IFN α_{2b} despite increased HBeAg seroconversion to 60% at 5-year follow-up.[48] Compared with IFN-based therapy, HBsAg seroclearance was almost negligible and only in HBeAg-positive patients after 1-year on Nuc therapy.[5] The 5-year HBsAg seroclearance rate increased to 6.4% of ETV-treated and 11% of TDF-treated HBeAg-positive patients, but still less than 1% in HBeAg-negative patients.[49]

SUMMARY AND PERSPECTIVES

Overall long-term data show that IFN-based therapy in HBeAg-positive patients results in cumulative HBeAg seroconversion, an increase in HBsAg seroclearance, and reduction of fibrosis/cirrhosis and/or the development of HCC, especially in patients with a sustained response. Of the HBeAg-negative patients, sustained responders and those who lost HBsAg have better outcomes. Because Peg IFN is more effective than conventional IFN in the treatment of chronic hepatitis B and may result in a sustained and delayed response, more long-term follow-up data will probably show that Peg IFNs have similar or even better effects.

Studies have also shown that maintained suppression of HBV replication by Nuc therapy may reduce the worsening of liver fibrosis, reverse advanced fibrosis, reduce the development of cirrhosis, and prevent further disease progression such as hepatic decompensation, development of HCC, or liver death in patients with advanced fibrosis or cirrhosis. Given the high genetic barrier to drug resistance, ETV or TDF is the preferred Nuc to show long-term benefit of Nuc therapy.

However, current therapies only reduce the risk of disease or slow disease progression; they do not prevent all adverse sequelae. Monitoring for HCC with ultrasonography and α-fetoprotein assay is mandatory to improve outcomes by increasing early detection and the chance of curative treatment.[50] The development of safe and affordable agents and the development of management strategies to improve sustained or maintained HBV suppression should be the ultimate goal in the management of chronic HBV infection.

ACKNOWLEDGMENTS

The authors thank the long-term grant support provided by Chang Gung Medical Research Fund (SMRPG1005, BMRPG380061) and the Prosperous Foundation, Taipei, Taiwan; and the excellent assistance of Ms Su-Chiung Chu.

REFERENCES

1. Liaw YF, Chu CM. Hepatitis B virus infection. Lancet 2009;373:582–92.
2. Liaw YF. Impact of hepatitis B therapy on the long-term outcome of liver disease. Liver Int 2011;31(Suppl 1):117–21.
3. Liaw YF, Kao JH, Piratvisuth T, et al. Asian-Pacific consensus statement on the management of chronic hepatitis B: a 2012 update. Hepatol Int 2012;6: 531–61.
4. Lok AS, McMahon BJ. Chronic hepatitis B: update 2009. Hepatology 2009;50: 661–2. Available at: http://www.aasld.org/practiceguidelines/Pages/default.aspx. Accessed June 5, 2013.
5. European Association for the Study of the Liver. EASL clinical practice guidelines: management of chronic hepatitis B virus infection. J Hepatol 2012;57: 167–85.
6. Lin SM, Sheen IS, Chien RN, et al. Long-term beneficial effect of interferon therapy in patients with chronic hepatitis B virus infection. Hepatology 1999;29:971–5.
7. Lau GK, Piratvisuth T, Luo KX, et al, Peginterferon Alfa-2a HBeAg-Positive Chronic Hepatitis B Study Group. Peginterferon Alfa-2a, lamivudine, and the combination for HBeAg-positive chronic hepatitis B. N Engl J Med 2005;352:2682–95.
8. Lampertico P, Del Ninno E, Vigano M, et al. Long-term suppression of hepatitis B e antigen-negative chronic hepatitis B by 24-month interferon therapy. Hepatology 2003;37:756–63.
9. Papatheodoridis GV, Petraki K, Cholongitas E, et al. Impact of interferon-alpha therapy on liver fibrosis progression in patients with HBeAg-negative chronic hepatitis B. J Viral Hepat 2005;12:199–206.
10. Fattovich G, Giustina G, Sanchez-Tapias J, et al. Delayed clearance of serum HBsAg in compensated cirrhosis B: relation to interferon alpha therapy and disease prognosis. European Concerted Action on Viral Hepatitis (EUROHEP). Am J Gastroenterol 1998;93:896–900.
11. Marcellin P, Bonino F, Lau GK, et al. Sustained response of hepatitis B e antigen-negative patients 3 years after treatment with peginterferon alpha-2a. Gastroenterology 2009;136:2169–79.
12. Dienstag JL, Goldin RD, Heathcote EJ, et al. Histological outcome during long-term lamivudine therapy. Gastroenterology 2003;124:105–17.
13. Hadziyannis SJ, Tassopoulos NC, Heathcote EJ, et al. Long-term therapy with adefovir dipivoxil for HBeAg-negative chronic hepatitis B for up to 5 years. Gastroenterology 2006;131:1743–51.
14. Liaw YF, Gane E, Leung N, et al. 2-Year GLOBE trial results: telbivudine is superior to lamivudine in patients with chronic hepatitis B. Gastroenterology 2009; 136:486–95.
15. Chang TT, Lai CL, Kew Yoon S, et al. Entecavir treatment for up to 5 years in patients with hepatitis B e antigen-positive chronic hepatitis B. Hepatology 2010; 51:422–30.
16. Marcellin P, Gane E, Buti M, et al. Regression of cirrhosis during treatment with tenofovir disoproxil fumarate for chronic hepatitis B: a 5-year open-label follow-up study. Lancet 2013;381:468–75.

17. Mommeja-Marin H, Mondou E, Blum MR, et al. Serum HBV DNA as a marker of efficacy during therapy for chronic HBV infection: analysis and review of the literature. Hepatology 2003;37:1309–19.

18. Lin SM, Yu ML, Lee CM, et al. Interferon therapy in HBeAg positive chronic hepatitis reduces cirrhosis and hepatocellular carcinoma. J Hepatol 2007;46:45–52.

19. Niederau C, Heintges T, Lange S, et al. Long-term follow-up of HBeAg-positive patients treated with interferon alfa for chronic hepatitis B. N Engl J Med 1996; 334:1422–7.

20. Brunetto MR, Oliveri F, Coco B, et al. Outcome of anti-HBe positive chronic hepatitis B in alpha-interferon treated and untreated patients: a long term cohort study. J Hepatol 2002;36:263–70.

21. Buster EH, Hansen BE, Buti M, et al. Peginterferon alpha-2b is safe and effective in HBeAg-positive chronic hepatitis B patients with advanced fibrosis. Hepatology 2007;46:388–94.

22. Chu CM, Liaw YF. Hepatitis B virus-related cirrhosis: natural history and treatment. Semin Liver Dis 2006;26:142–52.

23. Sung JJ, Tsoi KK, Wong VW, et al. Meta-analysis: treatment of hepatitis B infection reduces risk of hepatocellular carcinoma. Aliment Pharmacol Ther 2008;28: 1067–77.

24. Yang YF, Zhao W, Zhong YD, et al. Interferon therapy in chronic hepatitis B reduces progression to cirrhosis and hepatocellular carcinoma: a meta-analysis. J Viral Hepat 2009;16:265–71.

25. Miyake Y, Kobashi H, Yamamoto K. Meta-analysis: the effect of interferon on development of hepatocellular carcinoma in patients with chronic hepatitis B virus infection. J Gastroenterol 2009;44:470–5.

26. Wong GL, Yiu KK, Wong VW, et al. Meta-analysis: reduction in hepatic events following interferon-alfa therapy of chronic hepatitis B. Aliment Pharmacol Ther 2010;32:1059–68.

27. Marcellin P, Chang TT, Lim SG, et al. Long-term efficacy and safety of adefovir dipivoxil for the treatment of hepatitis B e antigen-positive chronic hepatitis B. Hepatology 2008;48:750–8.

28. Yuen MF, Seto WK, Chow DH, et al. Long-term lamivudine therapy reduces the risk of long-term complications of chronic hepatitis B infection even in patients without advanced disease. Antivir Ther 2007;12:1295–303.

29. Ono A, Suzuki F, Kawamura Y, et al. Long-term continuous entecavir therapy in nucleos(t)ide-naïve chronic hepatitis B patients. J Hepatol 2012;57:508–14.

30. Yokosuka O, Takaguchi K, Fujioka S, et al. Long-term use of entecavir in nucleoside-naïve Japanese patients with chronic hepatitis B infection. J Hepatol 2010;52:791–9.

31. Chang TT, Liaw YF, Wu SS, et al. Long-term entecavir therapy results in the reversal of fibrosis/cirrhosis and continued histological improvement in patients with chronic hepatitis B. Hepatology 2010;52:886–93.

32. Liaw YF, Sung JJY, Chow WC, on behalf of the CALM study group. Lamivudine for patients with chronic hepatitis B and advanced liver disease. N Engl J Med 2004;351:1521–31.

33. Kim CH, Um SH, Seo YS, et al. Prognosis of hepatitis B-related liver cirrhosis in the era of oral nucleos(t)ide analog antiviral agents. J Gastroenterol Hepatol 2012;27:1589–95.

34. Lampertico P, Viganò M, Manenti E, et al. Low resistance to adefovir combined with lamivudine: a 3-year study of 145 lamivudine-resistant hepatitis B patients. Gastroenterology 2007;133:1445–51.

35. Lampertico P, Soffredini R, Vigano M, et al. Entecavir treatment for Nuc naïve, field practice patients with chronic hepatitis B: excellent viral suppression and safety profile over 5 years of treatment. Hepatology 2012;56:370–71A (poster: 366).

36. Zoutendijk R, Reijnders JG, Zoulim F, et al. Virological response to entecavir is associated with a better clinical outcome in chronic hepatitis B patients with cirrhosis. Gut 2013;62(5):760–5.

37. Di Marco V, Marzano A, Lampertico P, et al, Italian Association for the Study of the Liver (AISF) Lamivudine Study Group, Italy. Clinical outcome of HBeAg-negative chronic hepatitis B in relation to virological response to lamivudine. Hepatology 2004;40:883–91.

38. Papatheodoridis GV, Lampertico P, Manolakopoulos S, et al. Incidence of hepatocellular carcinoma in chronic hepatitis B patients receiving nucleos(t)ide therapy: a systematic review. J Hepatol 2010;53:348–56.

39. Eun JR, Lee HJ, Kim TN, et al. Risk assessment for the development of hepatocellular carcinoma: according to on-treatment viral response during long-term lamivudine therapy in hepatitis B virus-related liver disease. J Hepatol 2010; 53:118–25.

40. Kurokawa M, Hiramatsu N, Oze T, et al. Long-term effect of lamivudine treatment on the incidence of hepatocellular carcinoma in patients with hepatitis B virus infection. J Gastroenterol 2012;47:577–85.

41. Papatheodoridis GV, Manolakopoulos S, Touloumi G, et al. Virological suppression does not prevent the development of hepatocellular carcinoma in HBeAg-negative chronic hepatitis B patients with cirrhosis receiving oral antiviral(s) starting with lamivudine monotherapy: results of the nationwide HEPNET. Greece cohort study. Gut 2011;60:1109–16.

42. Hosaka T, Suzuki F, Kobayashi M, et al. Long-term entecavir treatment reduces hepatocellular carcinoma incidence in patients with hepatitis B virus infection. Hepatology 2012. [Epub ahead of print]. http://dx.doi.org/10.1002/hep.26180.

43. Chen YC, Jeng WJ, Chien RN, et al. Hepatocellular carcinoma development in HBe-negative hepatitis B cirrhotic patients with Entecavir treatment. J Hepatol 2013;58:S214 (Posters 521).

44. Buti M, Fung S, Gane E, et al. Clinical, virological, serological and histological outcomes in cirrhotic patients with chronic hepatitis B (CHB) treated with tenofovir disoproxil fumarate (TDF) for up to 5 years. J Hepatol 2012;56:S197–8 (poster: 501).

45. Chu CM, Liaw YF. Hepatitis B surface antigen seroclearance during chronic HBV infection. Antivir Ther 2010;15:133–43.

46. Buster EH, Flink HJ, Cakaloglu Y, et al. Sustained HBeAg and HBsAg loss after long-term follow-up of HBeAg-positive patients treated with peginterferon alpha-2b. Gastroenterology 2008;135:459–67.

47. Marcellin P, Bonino F, Yurdaydin C, et al. Hepatitis B surface antigen levels: association with 5-year response to peginterferon alfa-2a in hepatitis B e-antigen-negative patients. Hepatol Int 2013;7(1):88–97.

48. Wong VW, Wong GL, Yan KK, et al. Durability of peginterferon alfa-2b treatment at 5 years in patients with hepatitis B e antigen-positive chronic hepatitis B. Hepatology 2010;51:1945–53.

49. Aghemo A, Lampertico P, Colombo M. Assessing long-term treatment efficacy in chronic hepatitis B and C: between evidence and common sense. J Hepatol 2012;57:1326–35.

50. Liaw YF. Prevention and surveillance of hepatitis B virus-related hepatocellular carcinoma. Semin Liver Dis 2005;25(Suppl 1):40–7.

Results of Treatment of Chronic Hepatitis B with Pegylated Interferon

Mauro Viganò, MD, PhD[a], Giampaolo Mangia, MD[b],
Pietro Lampertico, MD, PhD[b],*

KEYWORDS

- Chronic hepatitis B • Pegylated interferon • Sustained response • HBsAg levels
- IL28B polymorphism • HBV DNA

KEY POINTS

- Antiviral therapy of chronic hepatitis B patients is aimed to improve quality of life and survival by preventing progression of liver disease.
- To date, a course of PegIFN may be the most appropriate first line treatment strategy when the purpose of treatment is to achieve a sustained response after a defined treatment course compared with third-generation NUC requiring long-term administration.
- Despite the higher rates of off-therapy response of PegIFN compared with NUC, its benefits are restricted to a subgroup of patients only.
- To increase the rates of patients who may benefit from interferon-based treatment, minimizing the adverse events, a careful patient selection based on baseline features (ALT and HBV DNA levels, virus genotype and host genetic factors) or on treatment HBsAg kinetics are required for an individualized treatment optimization.

INTRODUCTION

Chronic infection with the Hepatitis B virus (HBV) represents major health problems worldwide, because roughly 400 million people are infected by virus.[1] Antiviral therapy of chronic hepatitis B (CHB) patients is aimed to improve quality of life and survival by preventing progression of liver damage to cirrhosis, hepatic decompensation, hepatocellular carcinoma, esophageal variceal bleeding, and death.[2–4] This goal can be achieved if HBV replication can be suppressed in a sustained or maintained manner

Financial Disclosure: M. Viganò: Speaking and Teaching: Roche, Gilead Sciences, BMS; P. Lampertico: Speaking bureau: BMS, Roche, Gilead Sciences, GSK.
[a] Hepatology Division, Ospedale San Giuseppe, Università degli Studi di Milano, Via San Vittore 12, Milano 20123, Italy; [b] 1st Division of Gastroenterology, "A.M. e A. Migliavacca" Center for the Study of Liver Disease, Fondazione IRCCS Cà Granda Ospedale Maggiore Policlinico, Università degli Studi di Milano, Via Francesco Sforza 35, Milano 20122, Italy
* Corresponding author.
E-mail address: pietro.lampertico@unimi.it

by either short-term "curative" treatment with interferon (IFN)-based treatment or long-term "suppressive" therapy with third-generation nucleot(s)ide analogues (NUCs), like entecavir (ETV) and tenofovir (TDF), that are the most potent and high barrier to resistance analogues, able to achieve a virologic suppression in most patients during the first 2 years of treatment. These drugs are well tolerated and have few side effects but require prolonged, probably lifelong, use because reactivation is common if treatment is stopped.[2–4] The main advantages of IFN over NUCs are the absence of resistance and the immunomodulatory properties that induce a direct inhibition of viral replication and the enhancement of the host's antiviral immune response (**Table 1**). This synergic effect may result in a sustained diseases remission in one-fourth of patients and a subsequent HBsAg seroclearance, which represent the ideal end point of any anti-HBV treatment, in a significant proportion of them.[5–7] Unfortunately, treatment with Pegylated-interferon (PegIFN) entails significant side effects and is contraindicated in some patient categories. The major hindrances to its wide use are the need for parenteral therapy and for the clinical and laboratory monitoring, its side-effects profile, and the lack of effectiveness in a large proportion of patients; therefore, PegIFN treatment is usually considered for young patients without contraindication, having mild to moderate fibrosis and willing to receive the drug.

INTERFERON
Alpha Interferons: Mechanisms of Action

Alpha interferons (IFN-α), belonging to IFN type I group, are naturally occurring intercellular signaling proteins that induce an antiviral state in cells and inhibit cellular proliferation and immunomodulation. Type I IFNs also include IFN-β and IFN-ω; 2 other types of IFN exist, type II and III, which include IFN-γ and IFN-λ.[8] The cellular activities of IFN-α are mediated by the products of the IFN-inducible genes. Subcutaneous administration of IFN-α triggers a complex intracellular cascade from IFN receptor via the JAK-STAT pathway that ultimately results in transcription of the so-called IFN-stimulated genes, a group of more than 30 genes directly responsible for IFN effects. The IFN-stimulated gene products include a double-stranded RNA-dependent protein kinase, which inhibits protein translation blocking elongation factor eIF2, and 2',5'-oligoadenylate synthase, an enzyme activating RNAse L, which in

	PegIFN	NUC
Pros	• Finite duration treatment • Absence of resistance • Higher rates of anti-HBe seroconversion and HBsAg loss with short-term treatment • Durable anti-HBe seroconversion • Immune-mediated control of HBV infection	• Potent HBV suppression • Good tolerance • Oral administration
Cons	• Moderate antiviral effect • Poor tolerability • Risk of side effects • Subcutaneous injection	• Indefinite duration • Risk of resistance • Unknown long-term safety • Increase cost over time • Low rates of HBsAg loss • Low durability anti-HBe seroconversion

Table 1
Pros and cons of pegylated interferon (PegIFN) versus nucleos(t)ide analogues (NUCs) for the treatment of chronic hepatic B (CHB)

turn mediates RNA degradation.[9] In addition to direct antiviral effects, IFN-α binds to immune cells, stimulating MHC class I expression and T-lymphocyte differentiation in T-helper type 1 phenotype, thus enhancing cellular immunity. Recent studies suggest a synergic role of natural immune response through activation of natural killer cells in viral clearance via enhanced cytotoxicity.[10] The result of these synergic effects is the induction of an "antiviral state" in infected cells through direct inhibition of viral replication and enhancement of the host's antiviral immune response.

Pharmacology of PegIFN

The efficacy of IFN-α therapy is hampered by protein characteristics and a suboptimal pharmacokinetic profile including poor stability, rapid absorption, a short half-life, large volume distribution, and rapid elimination via the kidney that ultimately determined wide fluctuations in serum concentrations and immunogenicity.[11] Thus, frequent dosing is required to achieve effective therapeutic concentrations in plasma and large fluctuations in serum concentrations occur resulting in peaks and troughs of drug concentration. Clinically this resulted in increased side effects after every administration of IFN and concomitant impaired suppression of viral replication when drug concentrations were waning.

Technology has enabled activation of the polyethylene glycol (Peg) moiety through substitution of the hydroxyl group by an electrophilic functional group. The reactive functional group of activated Peg can be attached to a specific site (ie, amine, sulphydryl group, or other nucleophile on the protein). Peg is an inert nontoxic polymer that can be used to modify the pharmacologic properties of biologically active proteins without completely inactivating their intrinsic biologic activity. The attachment of a Peg to the IFN (PegIFN) increases the half-life of the conjugated protein and decreases the renal clearance of a drug. Moreover, the pegylation process has the further benefit of creating a so-called "water cloud" effect that decreases antigenicity, immunogenicity, and proteolytic degradation of the native protein, ultimately determining a longer half-life of the pharmacologically active moiety.[12] Reduced clearance of PegIFN results in increased circulation time and sustained systemic exposure of the pegylated compound and this enables once-a-week dosing without wide fluctuations in serum concentrations. Overall, pegylation of the IFN-α molecule has provided substantial improvements in terms of side effects, adherence, and suppression of viral replication.[11,12] Two forms of PegIFN currently exist, PegIFNα2a and PegIFNα2b; both drugs share the same mechanism of action but show some differences in terms of efficacy as well as safety profile due to their peculiar pharmacokinetic and pharmacodynamic properties.[13] PegIFNα2b is not licensed for HBV treatment in most European countries.

Adverse Events of PegIFN

Treatment with PegIFN is associated with considerable adverse events (AE); the most frequently reported are a flulike syndrome, headache, myalgia, fatigue, and local reactions at the injection site.[5–7] These common AE are acceptable in most patients and typically present early during therapy, whereas neuropsychiatric side effects associated with PegIFN use, such as mood changes and irritability without depression, tend to present in the later stages. PegIFN has mild myelosuppressive effects leading to neutropenia and thrombocytopenia with clinically significant symptoms, including bleeding and infections, in only a select group of patients.[14]

Patients with decompensated cirrhosis have an absolute contraindication to PegIFN therapy, whereas in patients with advanced fibrosis/cirrhosis PegIFN therapy is generally well-tolerated and not contraindicated. However, the hepatitis flares, that have been reported to occur during and off treatment, may lead to hepatic decompensation.

On the other hand, PegIFN is contraindicated in patients receiving chemotherapy or immunosuppression, patients who are pregnant or willing to be pregnant, and all patients having some concomitant medical illness (ie, autoimmune disease, uncontrolled severe depression or psychosis, seizures, heart and lung disease). Close monitoring with clinical examinations and measurement of serum chemistries, complete blood counts, and thyroid function tests is required throughout therapy in all patients.

PEGIFN FOR HBEAG-POSITIVE PATIENTS
Registration Trials

In 2003, a trial of PegIFN showed benefit over conventional IFN in patients with HBeAg-positive CHB following treatment for 24 weeks. The combined response (ie, HBeAg loss, HBV DNA suppression, and alanine aminotransferase [ALT] normalization with PegIFNα-2a) was twice that achieved with conventional IFNα-2a (24% vs 12%, P = .036) with similar frequency and severity of AE.[15] In 2005, Lau and colleagues[5] investigated in 814 HBeAg-positive patients the efficacy of a 48-week course of PegIFNα-2a with and without the addition of lamivudine (LMV), in comparison with LMV alone. After 24 weeks of follow-up, significantly more patients who received PegIFNα-2a monotherapy or plus LMV than those who received LMV monotherapy had HBeAg seroconversion (32% vs 27% vs 19%, respectively) or HBV DNA levels less than 100,000 copies/mL (32% vs 34% vs 22%, respectively). Despite providing greater on-treatment HBV DNA suppression, the addition of LMV to PegIFN did not produce any advantage in terms of response rate 24 weeks posttreatment compared with PegIFN monotherapy. Moreover, 16 patients receiving PegIFNα-2a ± LMV had HBsAg seroconversion as compared with none in the group receiving LMV alone (P = .001) (**Fig. 1**). The rates of serious AE were similar in those treated with PegIFNα-2a ± LMV but were significantly less frequent in the group on LMV alone,

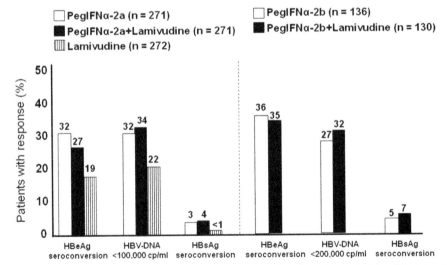

Fig. 1. Rates of virologic and serologic response 6 months after the end of PegIFN ± lamivudine treatment in HBeAg-positive patients enrolled in the 2 registration trials. (*Data from* Lau GK, Piratvisuth T, Luo KX, et al. Peginterferon Alfa-2a, lamivudine, and the combination for HBeAg-positive chronic hepatitis B. N Engl J Med 2005;352:2682–95; and Janssen HL, van Zonneveld M, Senturk H, et al. Pegylated interferon alfa-2b alone or in combination with lamivudine for HBeAg-positive chronic hepatitis B: a randomised trial. Lancet 2005;365:123–9.)

however, without significant differences between the rates of overall drugs discontinuation. Multivariate analysis indicated that response to PegIFN was associated with higher baseline ALT and lower HBV DNA and HBeAg levels, but not with gender, age, race, or body weight. Genotype A infection was associated with a better response (52%) compared with genotypes B (30%), C (31%), and D (22%).[5] In the long-term follow-up study of 150 Asian HBeAg-positive patients, originally enrolled in the Lau study, 58 (39%) achieved HBeAg seroconversion 6 months after the end of treatment (EOT), which was sustained after an additional 6 months of follow-up in 48 (83%) patients, whereas 14 of the 92 (15%) patients who lacked an HBeAg response at 6 months off-treatment achieved this end point in the further 6 months of follow-up. Overall, 12 months after the EOT, 41% of patients achieved HBeAg seroconversion with 79% and 38% of the patients having HBV DNA levels less than 100,000 and less than 400 copies/mL, respectively.[16]

In 2005 Janssen and colleagues[6] treated 266 HBeAg-positive patients for 52 weeks with PegIFNα-2b with LMV (n = 130) in comparison with PegIFNα-2b alone (n = 136). More patients in the PegIFNα-2b + LMV combination-therapy group than of the PegIFNα-2b monotherapy group had cleared HBeAg at the EOT (44% vs 29%, P = .01), although 26 weeks after EOT the rates of HBeAg seroclearance were similar (35% vs 36%) in the treatment groups. Similarly, at EOT, more patients in the combination-therapy than in the monotherapy group had HBV DNA suppression (i.e., less than 200,000 and 400 copies/mL [74% vs 29% and 33% vs 10%; $P<.0001$, respectively]) but again the rates of a sustained HBV DNA suppression were similar at the end of follow-up (32% vs 27% and 9% vs 7%; P = .44 and P = .43, respectively). Rates of HBsAg seroconversion were 7% and 5% in the 2 groups, respectively (see **Fig. 1**). Genotype A and B infection were associated with a higher rate of HBeAg loss (47% and 44%, respectively) at the end of follow-up compared with genotypes C and D (28% and 25%, respectively), whereas there was no difference in HBeAg loss according to HBV genotype between the 2 treatment groups. Multivariate analysis indicates that patients infected with HBV genotype A were more likely to respond to treatment than those with genotype D (odds ratio [OR] 2.4; 95% confidence interval [CI] 1.3–4.6, P = .01) or C (OR 3.6; 95%CI 1.4–8.9, P = .006), whereas patients with genotype B were slightly but not significantly more likely to respond than those with genotype C (OR 2.2; 95%CI 0.7–7.0, P = .18). Other baseline factors predictive of response were low viral load (OR 1.6; 95%CI 1.3–1.8, P = .009), high ALT concentrations (OR 1.1; 95%CI 1.0–1.2, P = .02), and absence of previous IFN therapy (OR 2.2; 95%CI 1.1–4.5, P = .04). Overall, the frequencies and severity of AE were similar for the treatment groups.

A representative cohort of 172 patients treated with PegIFNα-2b ± LMV in the aforementioned study was enrolled in a subsequent follow-up evaluation. Three years after treatment, HBeAg seroconversion was sustained in 70%; 37% and 11% of the patients were HBeAg and HBsAg seronegative, respectively, and among the initial responders HBeAg and HBsAg were lost in 81% and 30% of the patients, respectively.[17]

Recently, Liaw and colleagues,[18] in a controlled trial of 544 HBeAg-positive patients randomized to receive PegIFNα-2a 90 μg/wk or 180 μg/wk for 24 or 48 weeks, reported that the licensed PegIFNα-2a treatment regimen (180 μg weekly for 48 weeks) was the most efficacious and beneficial for HBeAg-positive patients compared with lower doses and shorter durations.

How to Optimize PegIFN Therapy in HBeAg-positive Patients?

Several strategies such as a de novo combination or sequential therapy with NUC, pretreatment or on-treatment selection of candidates at greater likelihood of response, have been implemented to increase the cost-effectiveness of PegIFN therapy.

On the assumption that the direct antiviral action of analogues may lower baseline HBV DNA levels and subsequently improve the immunomodulatory action of PegIFN leading to higher responses to PegIFN, this strategy was tested by several investigators. However, simultaneous commencement of PegIFN and LMV tends to provide more profound viral suppression without superior sustained virologic off-treatment response compared with PegIFN monotherapy.[5,6] In a multicenter prospective study, 160 HBeAg-positive patients were randomized to PegIFNα-2a monotherapy or to individualized combination therapy with PegIFNα-2a + adefovir dipivoxil (ADV) based on the baseline features and treatment response. At week 96, combined response (ALT normalization and HBV DNA undetectable), HBeAg clearance, and seroconversion rates were higher in those patients treated with the combination than with PegIFNα-2a alone.[19] A prospective, randomized, open-label study in HBeAg-positive patients compared the efficacy of the combination of PegIFNα-2a for 48 weeks plus 1.6 mg thymosin α-1 twice a week for the first 12 weeks to PegIFNα-2a for 48 weeks. The rates of the combined response, defined as HBeAg seroconversion, HBV DNA suppression, and ALT normalization, at the EOT and at the end of follow-up were similar among the combination and the monotherapy groups without significant differences in the observed AE.[20] A study in 159 HBeAg-positive patients reported that a combination of PegIFNα-2a with telbivudine (LdT) led to a higher rate of undetectable HBV viral load and greater reductions in HBeAg and HBsAg levels than either drug alone. However, the high risk of severe polyneuropathy development in those treated with the combination therapy has led to an early discontinuation of the study.[21] Thus, presently the combinations of PegIFN with LdT should be avoided.[2] One study investigated whether staggered commencement of PegIFN and LMV treatment has more potent virologic suppression than simultaneous regimes.[22] Thirty HBeAg-positive patients were randomized in a 1:1:1 ratio to 32-week PegIFN started simultaneously with LMV (group 1), 8 weeks before LMV (group 2) or 8 weeks after commencement of LMV (group 3). At week 52, HBeAg seroconversion developed in 6 patients in group 1, 3 patients in group 2, and 1 patient in group 3; however, at 24 weeks posttreatment, patients with sustained HBeAg seroconversion were similar among the 3 groups (5 vs 3 vs 4, respectively). In another study 36 treatment-naive HBeAg-positive patients who received LMV 100 mg per day for 4 weeks before adding PegIFN for the following 24 weeks achieved higher sustained virologic responses compared with the 27 patients who received PegIFN from the start.[23] Six months after therapy, undetectable HBV DNA and HBeAg losses were higher in the first group than in the latter group (50% vs 15%; $P = .028$; 39% vs 15%; $P = .05$, respectively). Recently, one study compared virologic response rates at week 48 (i.e., HBeAg loss with HBV DNA <200 IU/mL in 160 HBeAg-positive patients who received entecavir [ETV] 0.5 mg daily alone for 48 weeks or a 24-week addition of PegIFNα-2a 180 μg weekly after 24 weeks of ETV monotherapy).[24] Response was achieved in 18% of patients who received PegIFN add-on, compared with 8% of patients treated with ETV alone ($P = .07$), and the PegIFN add-on group showed higher HBsAg reduction compared with ETV alone (0.84 vs 0.32 $\log_{10}$ IU/mL, $P<.001$) with only one patient having HBsAg clearance belonging to the former group. In summary, all these studies comparing PegIFN + NUC combination therapy versus PegIFN monotherapy failed to provide convincing evidence for a superior efficacy of the former strategy.

Another possible approach to increase the cost-effectiveness of PegIFN is to select to treat only patients with a high probability of response. Low baseline HBV DNA, high ALT levels, younger age, female gender, and HBV genotype A and B are all well-known predictors of sustained responses. Unfortunately, viremia and ALT tend to fluctuate over time, making the prediction of response by these variables in a given patient rather cumbersome.[25]

In 115 HBeAg-positive patients treated with PegIFNα-2a for 6 to 12 months, HBV genotype, major sequences of precore stop codon/basal core promoter (BCP), and 3 single-nucleotide polymorphisms among the HLA-DPA1, HLA-DPB1, and IL28B regions were assessed.[26] HBeAg seroconversion 6 months off-therapy was achieved in 26% of the patients, without any difference between Thymine/Thymine and non-TT IL28B rs8099917 genotypes (26% vs 25%), as was the case for the combined off-treatment response defined as HBeAg seroconversion, HBV DNA less than 20,000 IU/mL, and ALT normalization (18% vs 17%). By multivariate analysis, BCP mutation (OR 8.04, 95%CI 2.00–32.28) and rs3077G/G HLA-DPA1 genotype (OR 3.49, 95%CI 1.12–10.84) were associated with a higher HBeAg seroconversion rate; BCP mutation (OR 9.28, 95%CI 1.92–44.99) and baseline viral load $<2 \times 10^6$ IU/mL (OR 4.78, 95%CI 1.37–16.69) were associated with a higher combined off-treatment response rate.

A retrospective, multicenter study in 205 HBeAg-positive patients treated with PegIFNα-2a $\pm$ LMV showed IL28B genotype to be significantly associated with HBeAg seroconversion at the EOT.[27] Fifty percent of patients with rs12979860 Cytosine/Cytosine genotype seroconverted to anti-HBe compared with 29% of Cytosine/Thymine and 10% of TT ($P = .001$) with an adjusted OR of 3.16 (95%CI 1.26–8.52, $P = .013$) for genotype AA versus AG/GG at rs12980275 after adjustment for HBV genotype, age, levels of HBV DNA and ALT, and combination therapy. IL28B genotype was also independently associated with an increased probability of HBeAg seroconversion during long-term follow-up: HBsAg seroconversion rates were 54%, 35%, and 20% in patients with genotype AA, AG, and GG (adjusted hazard ratio 2.14; 95%CI, 1.14–4.31; $P = .018$ for AA vs AG/GG by Cox regression analysis). Importantly, IL28B genotype was associated with HBsAg clearance (hazard ratio, 3.47 for AA vs AG/GG; 95% 95%CI: 1.04–13.48, $P = .042$).

One more study performed in China in 512 HBeAg-positive patients treated with PegIFNα-2a (plus NUC in 50% of the cases) for 12 months showed that virologic and serologic response 6 months after the EOT were lower among TT compared with non-TT IL28B rs8099917 SNPs (29% vs 52%, $P = .003$).[28]

Overall, having these 3 studies provided conflicting results on the relationship between IL28B polymorphisms and sustained response to PegIFN; this test should not be implemented into clinical practice until more studies are available.

Reports of HBsAg decline in HBeAg-negative and HBeAg-positive patients undergoing IFN-based therapy suggested the potential role of this marker for prediction of a treatment response.[29] HBsAg levels at the end of PegIFN treatment have been shown to be significantly lower in both HBeAg-positive and HBeAg-negative patients with a sustained virologic response.[30–32] Because a rapid on-treatment decline of HBsAg levels predicts a sustained response, HBsAg levels at 12 or 24 weeks after the beginning of treatment have been associated with the identification of nonresponders or for tailoring treatment duration in responders. The lack of a significant decline of HBsAg at week 12 of PegIFN is a strong negative predictor of response in HBeAg-positive patients, demonstrated by Sonneveld and colleagues,[33] who showed that no decline in HBsAg levels at week 12 of PegIFNa-2b $\pm$ LMV had a 3% chance of achieving a response (i.e., HBeAg loss with HBV DNA <10,000 copies/mL) 26 weeks after treatment only (97% negative predictive value [NPV]). The very high NPV for response of the lack of any HBsAg level decline at week 12 of treatment in patients treated with PegIFNα-2b was not confirmed in those treated with PegIFNα-2a. The retrospective analysis of the PegIFNα-2a registration trial demonstrated 18% of patients lacking a HBsAg decline at week 12 could achieve HBeAg loss and HBV DNA less than 2000 IU/mL 6 months after treatment (82% NPV).[34] Piratvisuth and colleagues[35] demonstrated that patients with low HBsAg levels (<1500 IU/mL) at weeks 12 and 24 of PegIFNα-2a treatment had 57% and 54% chances of HBeAg seroconversion 6 months after completing treatment, respectively. Response rates were significantly lower in patients with intermediate HBsAg levels, that is, 1500 to 20,000 IU/mL (32% and 26%, respectively) or HBsAg levels greater than 20,000 IU/mL (16% and 15%, respectively) (P<.0001 for <1500 IU/mL vs higher levels). The association of on-treatment HBsAg levels and sustained post-treatment response was confirmed by the NEPTUNE study,[18] where HBeAg seroconversion rates 6 months after treatment were significantly higher in patients with HBsAg less than 1500 IU/mL at weeks 12 and 24 (58% and 57%, respectively) compared with patients with HBsAg 1500 to 20,000 IU/mL (42% and 35%, respectively) or patients with HBsAg greater than 20,000 IU/mL that did not achieve sustained response and may therefore be considered for discontinuation of therapy.

Recently, Sonneveld and colleagues[36] evaluated the performance of 2 recently proposed stopping rules: the absence of a HBsAg decline from baseline to week 12 or 24 compared with a prediction rule that uses HBsAg levels of less than 1500 IU/mL and more than 20,000 IU/mL at week 12 or 24[33,35] in a pooled dataset of 803 HBeAg-positive patients infected with HBV genotypes A through D treated for 1 year with PegIFN ± LMV from 3 global randomized studies.[5,6,18] Patients with an HBsAg level less than 1500 IU/mL at week 12 or 24 achieved response in 45% and 46%, respectively, whereas patients without HBsAg decline at week 12 achieved a response in 14% compared with 6% of patients with HBsAg greater than 20,000 IU/mL, but performance varied across HBV genotype (**Table 2**). A stopping rule based on absence of a decline at week 12 was superior for patients infected with genotype A (NPV 88%) or D (NPV 98%), whereas an HBsAg level greater than 20,000 IU/mL better identified nonresponders with genotype B (NPV 92%) or C (NPV 99%). At week 24, nearly all patients with HBsAg greater than 20,000 IU/mL failed to achieve a response, irrespective of HBV genotype (NPV 98%) (**Fig. 2**). Based on this analysis, HBsAg greater than 20,000 IU/mL at week 12 cannot be used for genotype A, and genotype-specific stopping rules are required at week 12: no decline for genotype A and D and greater than 20,000 IU/mL for genotype B or C. Irrespective of HBV genotype, low response rates have been observed among those with HBsAg greater than 20,000 IU/mL at week 24 and for such patients discontinuation is indicated at week 24.

At present, on-treatment HBsAg kinetics is the best predictor of nonresponse to PegIFN and should be implemented in everyday clinical practice.

Table 2
Performance of stopping rules at week 12 varies by HBV genotype

Genotype	HBsAg >20,000 IU/mL		No HBsAg Decline	
	Response[a]	HBsAg Loss	Response[a]	HBsAg Loss
A (n = 98)	17%	10%	12%	0%
B (n = 199)	8%	0%	32%	0%
C (n = 377)	2%	0%	17%	1%
D (n = 105)	4%	3%	2%	2%

[a] Response was defined as HBeAg loss with HBV DNA <2000 IU/mL and/or HBsAg loss 6 months posttreatment.

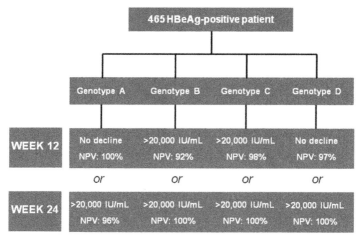

Fig. 2. Algorithm showing the chances of response defined as HBeAg loss with HBV DNA less than 2000 IU/mL and/or HBsAg loss 6 months posttreatment in 465 HBeAg-positive patients treated with PegIFN therapy, based on the presence of no HBsAg decline or HBsAg greater than 20,000 IU/mL at week 12 or 24. (*Data from* Sonneveld MJ, Hansen BE, Piratvisuth T, et al. Response-guided peginterferon therapy in HBeAg-positive chronic hepatitis B using serum hepatitis B surface antigen levels: a pooled analysis of 803 patients. Hepatology 2012;56:202A.)

PEGINT FOR HBEAG-NEGATIVE PATIENTS
Registration Trials

In 2004, a large multinational registration trial compared the virologic and biochemical response of 48 weeks of treatment with PegIFNα-2a ± LMV with LMV monotherapy in 537 HBeAg-negative patients.[7] After 24 weeks of follow-up, the percentage of patients with ALT normalization or HBV DNA levels less than 20,000 copies/mL was significantly higher among those treated with PegIFNα-2a ± LMV (60% and 44%; 59% and 43%, respectively) than with LMV alone (44% and 29%, respectively). The combination of PegIFNα-2a and LMV led to more profound EOT virologic response than PegIFNα-2a alone (92% vs 81%), yet the therapeutic effect was lost 6 months after treatment cessation when the rates decreased to 43% and 44%, respectively. Loss of HBsAg occurred in 12 patients in the PegIFNα-2a ± LMV groups as compared with none of the patients in the LMV group (**Fig. 3**). A subanalysis of patients treated with PegIFN ± LMV in Marcellin and colleagues study identified baseline high ALT, low HBV DNA levels, female gender, younger age, and HBV genotype as significant predictors of a combined response 24 weeks posttreatment.[37] In the PegIFN monotherapy arm, patients with genotype B or C had a greater chance of response than genotype D–infected patients ($P<.001$), the latter responding better to the combination with LMV than to PegIFN monotherapy ($P = .015$). In general, the HBV genotype was a strong predictor of the 1-year posttreatment response independent of LMV administration.

In the long-term follow-up study of 315 patients originally enrolled in the Marcellin study, the 3-year percentage of patients with normal ATL or with HBV DNA ≤10,000 copies/mL was higher for patients treated with PegIFN than with LMV (31% vs 18%; $P = .032$% and 28% vs 15% $P = .039$, respectively).[38] At year 5 of follow-up, 28 (12%) of the 230 patients treated with PegIFNα-2a ± LMV achieved HBsAg clearance, compared with 28% (20/72) in patients with HBV DNA ≤10,000 copies/mL 1 year posttreatment (**Fig. 4**).[39]

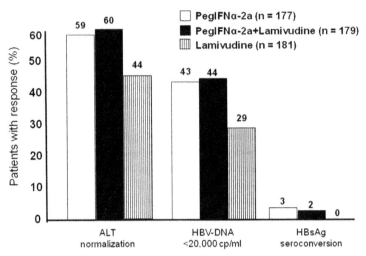

Fig. 3. Rates of biochemical, virologic, and serologic response 6 months after the end of PegIFN ± LMV treatment in HBeAg-negative patients enrolled in the Marcellin and colleagues registration trial. (*Data from* Marcellin P, Lau GK, Bonino F, et al. Peginterferon alfa-2a alone, lamivudine alone, and the two in combination in patients with HBeAg-negative chronic hepatitis B. N Engl J Med 2004;351:1206–17.)

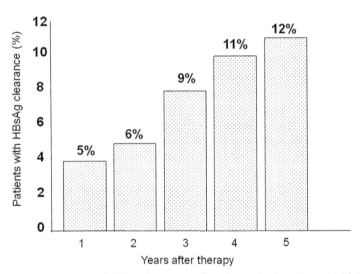

Fig. 4. Progressive increase of HBsAg loss rates after the end of treatment with PegIFN ± LMV in 230 HBeAg-negative patients. (*Data from* Piratvisuth T, Marcellin P, Brunetto M, et al. Sustained immune control 1 year post-treatment with Peginterferon Alfa-2a [40KD] (PEGASYS) is durable up to 5 years post-treatment and is associated with a high rate of HBsAg clearance in HBeAg-negative chronic hepatitis B. Presented at the 20th Conference of the Asian Pacific Association for the Study of the Liver (APASL). Beijing, China, March 25–28, 2010.)

How to Optimize PegIFN Treatment for HBeAg-Negative Patients?

To improve the virologic and serologic responses of PegIFN treatment in HBeAg-negative patients, several approaches have been developed.

A first strategy is to combine PegIFN with analogues on the assumption that the direct antiviral action of NUC may improve the immunomodulatory action of PegIFN. However, the addition of LMV to PegIFNα-2a, although leading to more profound end-of-treatment virologic response than PegIFN monotherapy, failed to improve sustained off-therapy response rates.[7]

An Italian multicenter study in 60 HBeAg-negative patients has shown similar sustained virologic response (i.e., HBV DNA <2000 IU/mL 24 weeks) after the EOT among those treated with a 48-week combination of PegIFNα-2a + ADV or PegIFNα-2a alone (23% vs 20%, $P = .75$) with only one patient (3%) in the combination group achieving HBsAg loss.[40] A pilot study that treated 20 consecutive HBeAg-negative patients with ADV for 20 weeks, then ADV + PegIFNα-2a for 4 weeks, and last with PegIFNα-2a for 44 weeks showed that 24 weeks after EOT 10 patients (50%) had serum HBV DNA less than 10,000 copies/mL.[41] One study that compared 48 weeks of PegIFNα-2a + Ribavirin (Rbv) or PegIFNα-2a alone showed that the addition of Rbv did not improve response (PARC trial). At 6 months after the EOT, the combined response (HBV DNA <10,000 copies/mL and normal ALT) was similar among the groups (20% vs 16%, $P = .49$), however, with higher risk of anemia and neutropenia in the combination therapy group.[42] Another study compared the efficacy and safety of 2 sequential regimens: PegIFN for 24 weeks followed by LdT for 24 weeks (PegIFN first) and or vice versa (LdT first) in 30 HBeAg-negative patients. At the end of follow-up (week 72), more patients treated with LdT first had HBV DNA less than 2000 IU/mL (47% vs 13%, $P = .046$). Sequential treatment with PegIFN followed or preceded by 24 weeks of LdT was safe; one only patient dropped out because of myalgia.[43] Currently, guidelines do not recommend the use of PegIFN in combination with NUC, but several studies are underway to assess whether such a combination is worth being pursued.[2]

A second approach to optimize therapy is to extend the length of PegIFN administration beyond 48 weeks, from previous studies showing that a 96-week course of standard IFN increases the sustained responses rates by reducing the risk of relapse.[44] In a pilot study from the United States, 7 HBeAg-negative patients received PegIFNα-2a for 60 weeks and 6 patients received PegIFNα-2a for 12 weeks followed by 48 weeks of PegIFNα-2a + LMV. Overall, sustained virologic response, defined as a reduction of serum HBV DNA of $\geq 2 \log_{10}$ copies/mL and HBV DNA less than 20,000 copies/mL at 24 week of follow-up, was achieved in 9 patients. This study concluded that 60 weeks of PegIFNα-2a ± LMV achieved a higher rate of response than historical controls treated with 48 weeks of PegIFN.[45] In a recent Italian multicenter study (PegBeLiver), 128 HBeAg-negative patients (mean age 45 years, 94% genotype D, 13% with cirrhosis) were randomized to weekly PegIFNα-2a 180 μg for 48 weeks (group A, n = 51), PegIFNα-2a 180 μg for 48 weeks, followed by PegIFNα-2a 135 μg weekly for an additional 48 weeks (group B, n = 52), or PegIFNα-2a 180 μg plus LMV (100 mg/day) for 48 weeks and then PegIFNα-2a 135 μg for 48 weeks (group C, n = 25).[46] At the EOT, virologic response (HBV DNA <2000 IU/mL) was similar among the groups (59%, 67%, and 72%), whereas the rates of virologic response observed 1 year after treatment were significantly higher in patients treated for 96 weeks (29% in group B, 12% in A and 20% in C, $P = .03$) (**Fig. 5**). Three patients in group B compared with none in group A and C became HBsAg negative (6% vs 0%) and 2 additional patients in group B had less than 10 IU/mL HBsAg levels compared with none in

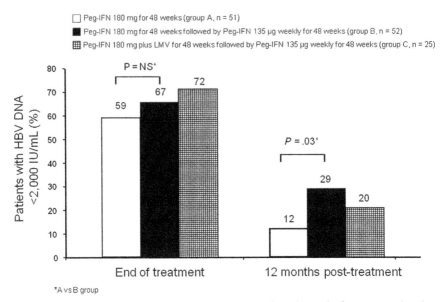

Fig. 5. Virologic response rates (HBV DNA <2000 IU/mL) at the end of treatment (EOT) and 12 months after EOT with PegIFN for 48 weeks (group A), PegIFN for 96 weeks (group B), and PegIFN + LMV for 48 weeks followed by PegIFN for 48 weeks (group C) in patients with HBeAg-negative chronic hepatitis B (PegBeLiver study). (*From* Lampertico P, Viganò M, Di Costanzo GG, et al. Randomised study comparing 48 and 96 weeks peginterferon a-2a therapy in genotype D HBeAg-negative chronic hepatitis B. Gut 2013;62:290–8.)

group A and C. Extended treatment was well tolerated without an increase in either the AE or the discontinuation rates compared with patients treated for 48 weeks.

An additional approach to optimize PegIFN therapy is to select patients according to pretreatment predictors, such as viral genotype and IL28B polymorphisms, and/or on-treatment predictors, such as HBsAg kinetics. HBeAg-negative patients infected with A through C viral genotypes do respond better to PegIFN therapy compared with genotype D patients (i.e., 50% vs 20%).[25] For other genotypes such as E, F and G, however, no studies are available yet.

Genomic studies would have the advantage to select patients according to a variable which, at variance from ALT and HBV DNA levels, is stable over time. The only existing data in HBeAg-negative patients come from 101 subjects treated with either conventional IFN or PegIFNα-2a for 24 months and followed up for 11 years after treatment.[47] Patients with IL28B rs12979860 genotype CC were shown to have higher EOT (69% vs 45%, P = .01) and higher sustained virologic response (31% vs 13%, P = .02) than non-CC patients. Interestingly, CC patients had a higher cumulative probability of clearing HBsAg during an observation period of 16 years (38% vs 12%, P = .039), a finding that was confirmed by multivariate analysis. The IL28B genotype was shown to be an independent predictor of both virologic and serologic responses together with low baseline HBV DNA levels, high ALT levels, and the duration of IFN therapy. To identify any possible association between IL28B polymorphisms and HBV genotype further, data in 93 genotype D patients were reanalyzed with IL28B stratification and showed 48% with CC, 41% with CT, and 11% with TT genotypes. The rates of EOT response, sustained virological response, and HBsAg clearance were still significantly higher in CC than in non-CC carriers (ie, 69% vs

44% [*P* = .014], 31% vs 12% [*P* = .028], and 29% vs 12% [*P* = .048]). When the assessment of the IL28B polymorphism was extended to include rs8099917, which was recently shown to improve the prediction of a response to PegIFN/Rbv therapy in chronic hepatitis C patients with the CT genotype of rs12979860, the favorable rs8099917 TT genotype was found in 100% of the rs12979860 CC patients compared with 31% of CT and 10% of TT patients only. The 42 rs12979860 CT patients with the rs8099917 TT genotype had a significantly higher rate of SVR and HBsAg seroclearance (23% vs 3%, *P* = .045 and 23% vs 0%, *P* = .007, respectively),[48] suggesting that multiple IL28B polymorphisms may be required to define the pretreatment probability of a virologic response at an individual level.

Several recent studies have looked at on-treatment HBsAg levels to predict response to PegIFN. In a landmark study of 48 HBeAg-negative patients receiving PegIFNα-2a, Moucari and colleagues[30] have reported that early on-therapy serologic (HBsAg) response could predict an SVR. A decline of 0.5 and 1 log IU/mL of serum HBsAg levels at weeks 12 and 24 of therapy, respectively, had a 90% NPV and a 89% positive predictive value for week 12 and a 97% NPV and a 92% positive predictive value for week 24 for the detection of patients who would achieve an SVR. After a retrospective analysis of serum HBsAg levels in the PegIFNα-2a registration study, patients who achieved a decline of ≥10% in serum HBsAg from baseline at 12 weeks of treatment had a higher probability of SVR than those with a less than 10% decline (47% vs 16%, *P*<.01).[49] The pattern of HBsAg decline in genotype D patients, who were underrepresented in this study, was investigated in Italy for the relationship between on-treatment HBsAg decline ≥10% and an SVR to PegIFN.[35] A ≥10% decline of HBsAg at week 24, but not at week 12 of treatment, was significantly associated with an SVR to PegIFN administered for 96 weeks only.[50] The absolute HBsAg level during treatment may also predict the response to IFN. One-third of the HBeAg-negative patients with HBsAg levels ≤1500 IU/mL at week 12 of PegIFNα-2a ± LMV cleared HBsAg 4 years after treatment compared with 4% of those with HBsAg greater than 1500 IU/mL (*P*<.001).[51] Brunetto and colleagues[31] showed that either an EOT serum HBsAg level less than 10 IU/mL or an on-treatment reduction greater than 2 $\log_{10}$ from baseline at week 48 was significantly associated with HBsAg loss in the next 3 years. On-treatment HBsAg levels may also help identify patients with a low probability of achieving SVR, leading to PegIFN withdrawal before the EOT is achieved.

A combination of a lack of decrease in HBsAg and less than 2 $\log_{10}$ IU/mL reduction in HBV DNA at week 12 predicts nonresponse in genotype D HBeAg-negative patients treated with PegIFNα-2a.[52,53] In 102 HBeAg-negative patients treated with PegIFNα-2a ± Rbv for 12 months, none of the 20 patients with unmodified HBsAg levels and a less than 2 $\log_{10}$ copies/mL decrease in HBV DNA had a long-term response defined as serum HBV DNA less than 10,000 copies/mL and normal ALT 6 months after the end of treatment (NPV = 100%) (**Fig. 6**).[52] This stopping rule has been recently confirmed in genotype D patients enrolled in the original PARC trial (n = 81) and in a validation dataset (n = 91) that also included patients treated with PegIFNα-2a for more than 48 weeks (**Fig. 7**).[53] This stopping rule, which was effective in both studies (*P* = .001), had a NPV of 100% in genotype D patients so that therapy could be discontinued in 19% of patients while all patients with an SVR were kept on treatment. Also, none of the 7 (21%) patients with unmodified HBsAg levels and less than 2 $\log_{10}$ HBV DNA decline at week 12 treated for 96 weeks achieved an SVR. These studies provide the rationale for stopping PegIFN at week 12 in approximately 20% of HBeAg-negative patients with a less than 2 $\log_{10}$ HBV DNA decline and no change in HBsAg levels, as these patients have no chance of achieving an SVR even if therapy is extended beyond week 48.

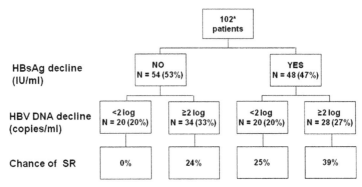

Fig. 6. Algorithm showing the chances of sustained response based on HBsAg decline and HBV DNA decline ≥2 log copies/mL at week 12 versus the baseline in HBeAg negative patients. (*Data from* Rijckborst V, Hansen BE, Cakaloglu Y, et al. Early on-treatment prediction of response to peginterferon alfa-2a for HBeAg-negative chronic hepatitis B using HBsAg and HBV DNA levels. Hepatology 2010;52:454–61.)

To optimize the outcome of PegIFN treatment further in HBeAg-negative, genotype D patients, a second stopping rule at week 24 has been proposed. Patients with HBsAg greater than 7500 IU/mL at week 24 had a very low chance (4%) of achieving a sustained response, defined as HBV DNA less than 2000 IU/mL 1 year

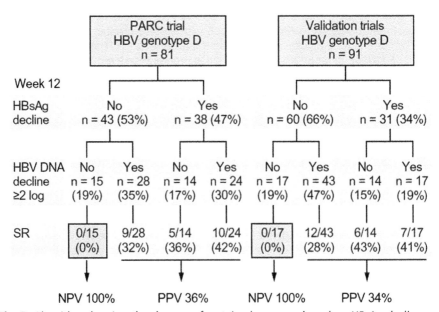

Fig. 7. Algorithm showing the chances of sustained response based on HBsAg decline and HBV DNA decline ≥2 log copies/mL at week 12 versus the baseline, in the validation study. (*Data from* Rijckborst V, Hansen BE, Ferenci P, et al. Validation of a stopping rule at week 12 using HBsAg and HBV DNA for HBeAg-negative patients treated with peginterferon alfa-2a. J Hepatol 2012;56:1006–11.)

after PegIFN treatment (NPV: 93% and 100% for 48 and 96 weeks treatment, respectively).[54] If externally validated, the 24-week cutoff might be a second stopping rule for PegIFNα-2a-treated patients, however, restricting patients infected with genotype D of HBV.

In summary, the best strategy to increase the cost-effectiveness of PegIFN therapy in HBeAg-negative patients is based on a week 12 stopping rule, which, however, requires full validation for non-genotype D–infected patients.

PEGIFN TREATMENT IN NUC RESPONDERS

Because it has been observed that during effective NUC therapy HBsAg decline is very slow and may require decades to achieve undetectable levels, an alternative use of PegIFN in CHB patients is to add on PegIFN to NUC responders to accelerate the HBsAg decline, induce seroclearance, and therefore discontinue any treatment.

One study reported HBsAg kinetics in 12 patients (9 HBeAg-negative) having undetectable HBV DNA (<116 copies/mL) for more than 6 months on NUCs (LMV = 1, LMV + ADV = 2, ETV = 7, ETV + TDF = 2) who additionally received PegIFN as an individualized therapy. After add on of PegIFN, a rapid decline of HBsAg occurred in 2 patients to HBsAg levels of 0.14 and 0.02 IU/mL at week 48, respectively (corresponding to a maximal reduction of 2.9 $\log_{10}$ and 4.25 $\log_{10}$). Three patients discontinued PegIFN early due to side effects, whereas 7 patients withdrew from treatment after a mean of 16 weeks due to a suboptimal HBsAg response (decline of 0.09 $\log_{10}$ only).[55]

A second study reported HBsAg kinetics in 10 HBeAg-negative patients having HBV DNA below the detection limit for more than 3 years on NUCs treatments (LMV = 1, ADV = 3, ETV = 2, LMV + ADV = 2, ADV + ETV = 2).[56] Four patients had a continuous decline of HBsAg to less than 10 IU/mL between weeks 24 and 48 and stopped all antiviral therapy and achieved HBsAg seroclearance that remained sustained 24 weeks after cessation of therapy and one had HBsAg seroconversion. In 5 of the 6 remaining patients, HBsAg levels highly decreased.

In a third study 12 HBeAg-negative patients with undetectable serum HBV DNA and stable HBsAg levels received 6 to 12 months of add-on PegIFN. HBsAg levels initially increased from 841 IU/mL to 1115 IU at month 1 and 927 IU at month 3, but later declined to 740, 634, and 509 IU at month 4, 5, and 6. Overall, HBsAg declined by approximately 50% within 6 months with 2 patients (20%) achieving HBsAg level less than 100 IU (78 and 13 IU). During an additional 3 months, 4 patients showed a further decline of HBsAg levels, from 951 to 221 IU/mL.[57]

Although these studies showed inconclusive results, because it is possible that HBsAg kinetics may have been higher with prolongation of therapy, the add-on concept merits being evaluated in a clinical trial, including more long-term responders to NUC therapy.

SUMMARY

Despite the improvement of antiviral treatment armamentarium, management of CHB patients remains complex in relation to the choice of the 2 different possible strategies: PegIFN versus NUCs. To date, a course of PegIFN may be the most appropriate first-line treatment strategy when the purpose of treatment is to achieve a sustained response after a defined treatment course compared with NUC requiring long-term administration. Despite the tolerability and the higher rates of off-therapy response compared with NUC, its benefits are restricted to a subgroup of patients only. To increase the rates of patients who may benefit from this treatment minimizing the adverse events, a careful patient selection and individualized treatment decisions to achieve a treatment optimization are required. In this decision-making process, all relevant factors for each individual patient should be accounted for balancing the potential risks and benefits. High ALT levels, low HBV DNA, virus genotype, and host genetic factors have been identified as pretreatment predictors of a response. However, these parameters have limited applicability in clinical practice because ALT and HBV DNA levels are time-dependent, whereas HBV genotype or IL28B SNPs require a specific test, not available in everyday clinical practice of a nonreferral center. To overcome this limitation, a response-guided therapy approach based on HBsAg levels (HBsAg >20,000 IU/mL at week 24 of treatment in HBeAg-positive patients and unmodified HBsAg levels plus <2 $\log_{10}$ HBV DNA decline at week 12 in HBeAg-negative patients) allow for the identification of nonresponders who can stop PegIFN.

REFERENCES

1. World Health Organization. Hepatitis B. World Health Organization fact sheet 204 (Revised August 2008). World Health Organization; 2008. Ref Type: Online Source. Available at: www.who.int/mediacentre/factsheets/fs204/en/.
2. European Association For The Study Of The Liver. EASL clinical practice guidelines: management of chronic hepatitis B virus infection. J Hepatol 2012;57: 167–85.
3. Lok AS, McMahon BJ. Chronic hepatitis B. Hepatology 2007;45:507–39.
4. Liaw YF, Kao JH, Piratvisuth T, et al. Asian-Pacific consensus statement on the management of chronic hepatitis B: a 2008 update. Hepatol Int 2012;6: 531–61.
5. Lau GK, Piratvisuth T, Luo KX, et al. Peginterferon Alfa-2a, lamivudine, and the combination for HBeAg-positive chronic hepatitis B. N Engl J Med 2005;352: 2682–95.
6. Janssen HL, van Zonneveld M, Senturk H, et al. Pegylated interferon alfa-2b alone or in combination with lamivudine for HBeAg-positive chronic hepatitis B: a randomised trial. Lancet 2005;365:123–9.
7. Marcellin P, Lau GK, Bonino F, et al. Peginterferon alfa-2a alone, lamivudine alone, and the two in combination in patients with HBeAg-negative chronic hepatitis B. N Engl J Med 2004;351:1206–17.
8. Platanias LC. Mechanisms of type-I- and type-II-interferon-mediated signalling. Nat Rev Immunol 2005;5:375–86.
9. Feld JJ, Hoofnagle JH. Mechanism of action of interferon and ribavirin in treatment of hepatitis C. Nature 2005;436:967–72.
10. Oliviero B, Mele D, Degasperi E, et al. Early NK cell activation predicts successful treatment outcome in chronic HCV infection. Dig Liver Dis 2011;43:S86.
11. Caliceti P. Pharmacokinetics of pegylated interferons: what is misleading? Dig Liver Dis 2004;36:S334–9.
12. Harris JM, Martin NE, Modi M. Pegylation: a novel process for modifying pharmacokinetics. Clin Pharmacokinet 2011;40:539–51.
13. Aghemo A, Rumi MG, Colombo M. Pegylated interferons alpha2a and alpha2b in the treatment of chronic hepatitis C. Nat Rev Gastroenterol Hepatol 2010;7: 485–94.
14. van Zonneveld M, Flink HJ, Verhey E, et al. The safety of pegylated interferon alpha-2b in the treatment of chronic hepatitis B: predictive factors for dose reduction and treatment discontinuation. Aliment Pharmacol Ther 2005;21: 1163–71.

15. Cooksley WG, Piratvisuth T, Lee SD, et al. Peginterferon alpha-2a (40 kDa): an advance in the treatment of hepatitis B e antigen-positive chronic hepatitis B. J Viral Hepat 2003;10:298–305.
16. Piratvisuth T, Lau G, Chao YC, et al. Sustained response to peginterferon alfa-2a (40 kD) with or without lamivudine in Asian patients with HBeAg-positive and HBeAg-negative chronic hepatitis B. Hepatol Int 2008;2:102–10.
17. Buster EH, Flink HJ, Cakaloglu Y, et al. Sustained HBeAg and HBsAg loss after long-term follow-up of HBeAg-positive patients treated with peginterferon alpha-2b. Gastroenterology 2008;135:459–67.
18. Liaw YF, Jia JD, Chan HL, et al. Shorter durations and lower doses of peginterferon alfa-2a are associated with inferior hepatitis B e antigen seroconversion rates in hepatitis B virus genotypes B or C. Hepatology 2011;54:1591–9.
19. Wang YD, Zhao CY, Wang W, et al. Improved efficacy by individualized combination therapy with Peg IFN-a 2a and ADV in HBeAg positive chronic hepatitis B patients. Hepatogastroenterology 2012;59:680–6.
20. Kim BH, Lee YJ, Kim W, et al. Efficacy of thymosin α-1 plus peginterferon α-2a combination therapy compared with peginterferon α-2a monotherapy in HBeAg-positive chronic hepatitis B: a prospective, multicenter, randomized, open-label study. Scand J Gastroenterol 2012;47:1048–55.
21. Marcellin P, Avila C, Wursthorn K, et al. Telbivudine (LdT) plus peg-interferon (Peg-IFN) in HBeAg-positive chronic hepatitis B: very potent antiviral efficacy but risk of peripheral neuropathy (PN). J Hepatol 2010;51:S6–7.
22. Chan HL, Wong VW, Chim AM, et al. Virological response to different combination regimes of peginterferon alpha-2b and lamivudine in hepatitis B e antigen positive chronic hepatitis B. Antivir Ther 2007;12:815–23.
23. Sarin SK, Sood A, Kumar M, et al. Effect of lowering HBV DNA levels by initial antiviral therapy before adding immunomodulator on treatment of chronic hepatitis B. Am J Gastroenterol 2007;102:96–104.
24. Sonneveld MJ, Xie Q, Zhang NP, et al. Adding peginterferon alfa-2a to entecavir increases HBsAg decline and HBeAg clearance - first results from a global randomized trial (ARES study). Hepatology 2012;56:199A.
25. Viganò M, Lampertico P. Antiviral drugs for HBV liver disease. Expert Opin Biol Ther 2011;11:285–300.
26. Tseng TC, Yu ML, Liu CJ, et al. Effect of host and viral factors on hepatitis B e antigen-positive chronic hepatitis B patients receiving pegylated interferon alpha-2a therapy. Antivir Ther 2011;16:629–37.
27. Sonneveld MJ, Wong VW, Woltman AM, et al. Polymorphisms near IL28B and serologic response to peginterferon in HBeAg-positive patients with chronic hepatitis B. Gastroenterology 2012;142:513–20.
28. Wu X, Xin Z, Zhu X, et al. Evaluation of susceptibility locus for response to interferon alpha based therapy in chronic hepatitis B patients in Chinese. Antiviral Res 2011;94:272–5.
29. Viganò M, Lampertico P. Clinical implications of HBsAg quantification in patients with chronic hepatitis B. Saudi J Gastroenterol 2012;18:81–6.
30. Moucari R, Mackiewicz V, Lada O, et al. Early serum HBsAg drop: a strong predictor of sustained virological response to pegylated interferon alfa-2a in HBeAg-negative patients. Hepatology 2009;49:1151–7.
31. Brunetto MR, Moriconi F, Bonino F, et al. Hepatitis B virus surface antigen levels: a guide to sustained response to peginterferon alfa-2a in HBeAg-negative chronic hepatitis B. Hepatology 2009;49:1141–50.

32. Wong VW, Wong GL, Yan KK, et al. Durability of peginterferon alfa-2b treatment at 5 years in patients with hepatitis B e antigen-positive chronic hepatitis B. Hepatology 2010;51:1945–53.

33. Sonneveld MJ, Rijckborst V, Boucher CA, et al. Prediction of sustained response to peginterferon alfa-2b for hepatitis B e antigen-positive chronic hepatitis B using on-treatment hepatitis B surface antigen decline. Hepatology 2010;52:1251–7.

34. Piratvisuth T, Marcellin P. Further analysis is required to identify an early stopping rule for peginterferon therapy that is valid for all hepatitis B e antigen-positive patients. Hepatology 2011;53:1054–5.

35. Piratvisuth T, Marcellin P, Popescu M, et al. Hepatitis B surface antigen: association with sustained response to peginterferon alfa-2a in hepatitis B e antigen-positive patients. Hepatol Int 2011. [Epub ahead of print].

36. Sonneveld MJ, Hansen BE, Piratvisuth T, et al. Response-guided peginterferon therapy in HBeAg-positive chronic hepatitis B using serum hepatitis B surface antigen levels: a pooled analysis of 803 patients. Hepatology 2012;56:202A.

37. Bonino F, Marcellin P, Lau GK, et al. Predicting response to peginterferon alpha-2a, lamivudine and the two combined for HBeAg-negative chronic hepatitis B. Gut 2007;56:699–705.

38. Marcellin P, Bonino F, Lau GK, et al. Sustained response of hepatitis B e antigen-negative patients 3 years after treatment with peginterferon alpha-2a. Gastroenterology 2009;136:2169–79.

39. Piratvisuth T, Marcellin P, Brunetto M, et al. Sustained immune control 1 year post-treatment with Peginterferon Alfa-2a [40KD] (PEGASYS) is durable up to 5 years post-treatment and is associated with a high rate of HBsAg clearance in HBeAg-negative chronic hepatitis B. Presented at the 20th Conference of the Asian Pacific Association for the Study of the Liver (APASL). Beijing, China, March 25–28, 2010.

40. Piccolo P, Lenci I, Demelia L, et al. A randomized controlled trial of pegylated interferon-alpha2a plus adefovir dipivoxil for hepatitis B e antigen negative chronic hepatitis B. Antivir Ther 2009;14:1165–74.

41. Moucari R, Boyer N, Ripault MP, et al. Sequential therapy with adefovir dipivoxil and pegylated interferon alfa-2a for HBeAg-negative patients. J Viral Hepat 2011;18:580–6.

42. Rijckborst V, Ter Borg MJ, Cakaloglu Y, et al. A randomized trial of peginterferon alpha-2a with or without ribavirin for HBeAg-negative chronic hepatitis B. Am J Gastroenterol 2010;105:1762–9.

43. Piccolo P, Lenci I, di Paolo D, et al. A randomized controlled trial of sequential peginterferon-alpha and telbivudine or vice versa for 48 weeks in HBeAg-negative chronic hepatitis B. Antivir Ther 2013;18(1):57–64. http://dx.doi.org/10.3851/IMP2281.

44. Lampertico P, Del Ninno E, Manzin A, et al. A randomized, controlled trial of a 24-month course of interferon alfa 2b in patients with chronic hepatitis B who had hepatitis virus DNA without hepatitis B e antigen in serum. Hepatology 1997;26:1621–5.

45. Gish RG, Lau DT, Schmid P, et al. A pilot study of extended duration peginterferon alfa-2a for patients with hepatitis B e antigen-negative chronic hepatitis B. Am J Gastroenterol 2007;102:2718–23.

46. Lampertico P, Viganò M, Di Costanzo GG, et al. Randomised study comparing 48 and 96 weeks peginterferon α-2a therapy in genotype D HBeAg-negative chronic hepatitis B. Gut 2013;62:290–8.

47. Lampertico P, Viganò M, Cheroni C, et al. IL28B polymorphisms predict interferon-related HBsAg seroclearance in genotype D HBeAg negative patients with chronic hepatitis B. Hepatology 2013;57(3):890–6. http://dx.doi.org/10.1002/hep.25749.

48. Lampertico P, Galmozzi E, Colombo M. Studies of IL28B genotype and response to peginterferon in chronic hepatitis B should be stratified by HBV genotype. Hepatology 2013;57(3):1283–4. http://dx.doi.org/10.1002/hep.25882.

49. Marcellin P, Piratvisuth T, Brunetto M, et al. On-treatment decline in serum HBsAg levels predicts sustained immune control 1 year posttreatment, subsequent HBsAg clearance in HBeAg-negative hepatitis B virus-infected patients treated with peginterferon alfa-2a. Hepatol Int 2010;4:151.

50. Lampertico P, Viganò M, Galeota Lanza A, et al. PegBeLiver study: HBsAg decline at week 24 of extended peginterferon alfa-2a (Peg-IFNa-2a) therapy is significantly associated with post-treatment response in HBeAg-negative genotype D patients. J Hepatol 2011;54:S293.

51. Marcellin P, Brunetto M, Bonino F, et al. In patients with HBeAg-negative chronic hepatitis B HBsAg serum levels early during treatment with peginterferon alfa-2a predict HBsAg clearance 4 years post-treatment. Hepatology 2008;48:718A.

52. Rijckborst V, Hansen BE, Cakaloglu Y, et al. Early on-treatment prediction of response to peginterferon alfa-2a for HBeAg-negative chronic hepatitis B using HBsAg and HBV DNA levels. Hepatology 2010;52:454–61.

53. Rijckborst V, Hansen BE, Ferenci P, et al. Validation of a stopping rule at week 12 using HBsAg and HBV DNA for HBeAg-negative patients treated with peginterferon alfa-2a. J Hepatol 2012;56:1006–11.

54. Lampertico P, Viganò M, Di Costanzo GG, et al. A response guided approach to peg-interferon alfa-2a at weeks 12 and 24 improves response rates in HBeAg-negative, genotype D chronic hepatitis B patients. Hepatology 2011;54:1021A.

55. Kittner JM, Sprinzl MF, Grambihler A, et al. Adding pegylated interferon to a current nucleos(t)ide therapy leads to HBsAg seroconversion in a subgroup of patients with chronic hepatitis B. J Clin Virol 2012;54:93–5.

56. Ouzan D, Penaranda G, Joly H, et al. Add-on of Peg interferon to a stable nucleoside regimen led to loos of HBsAg in chronic hepatitis HBeAg-negative patients. Hepatology 2011;54:1015A.

57. Lampertico P, Invernizzi F, Soffredini R, et al. Add-on Peg-IFN improves HBsAg kinetics in patients long-term fully suppressed by nucleos(t)ide analogs. J Hepatol 2012;56:S2–207.

Long-term Results of Treatment with Nucleoside and Nucleotide Analogues (Entecavir and Tenofovir) for Chronic Hepatitis B

Tarik Asselah, MD, PhD[a,b],*, Patrick Marcellin, MD, PhD[a,b]

KEYWORDS

- Personalized medicine • PEG-IFN • Analogues • Cirrhosis • Fibrosis regression

KEY POINTS

- Several antiviral therapies are available in the United States and Europe, including interferon-α, peginterferon-α-2a, lamivudine, adefovir dipivoxil, telbivudine, tenofovir, and entecavir.
- The treatment goal with analogues for chronic hepatitis B virus infection is the achievement of sustained suppression of viral replication with the aim to reduce the progression to cirrhosis and/or hepatocellular carcinoma, to prevent hepatic decompensation, and ultimately to improve survival.
- De novo monotherapy with an agent that has a high genetic barrier to resistance, such as entecavir or tenofovir, is recommended.
- Both entecavir and tenofovir have demonstrated considerable improvements in liver histology within long-term studies.
- For patients with mild disease, the treatment can be delayed with regular follow-up.

TREATMENT OBJECTIVE

The treatment goal for chronic hepatitis B virus (HBV) infection is the achievement of sustained suppression of viral replication with the aim to reduce the progression to cirrhosis and/or hepatocellular carcinoma (HCC), to prevent hepatic decompensation, and ultimately to improve survival.[1]

In a prospective, community-based, long-term study involving a cohort of 3653 HBsAg-positive individuals from Taiwan, a relationship was found between serum

[a] INSERM, U-773, CRB3; [b] Department of Hepatology, Service d'Hépatologie, Hôpital Beaujon, AP-HP, Université Paris-Diderot, 100 Boulevard du Général Leclerc, 92110 Clichy, France
* Corresponding author. INSERM U 481, Hôpital Beaujon, 100 Boulevard du Général Leclerc, Clichy 92110, France.
E-mail address: tarik.asselah@bjn.aphp.fr

Clin Liver Dis 17 (2013) 445–450
http://dx.doi.org/10.1016/j.cld.2013.05.001
1089-3261/13/$ – see front matter © 2013 Elsevier Inc. All rights reserved.

HBV DNA level and the risk of HCC.[2] The cumulative risk of HCC increased from 1.3% to 14.9% for HBV DNA levels of less than 300 copies/mL and $\geq 10^6$ copies/mL, respectively. Moreover, reduction of serum HBV DNA levels over time was associated with a 6-fold reduction in risk of HCC. Taken together, these data suggest that patients with ongoing HBV DNA replication have a higher risk for disease progression and may benefit from anti-HBV therapy. However, these studies do not define the level of replication clearly above which the risk of progression is increased. Long-term studies with sequential assessments of HBV DNA levels and liver histologic assessment are needed.

IMPROVED TREATMENT EFFICACY

In recent years, marked progress has been made in the treatment of chronic hepatitis B; several agents are currently approved and their efficacy has been evaluated in randomized controlled trials and long-term follow-up cohort studies: IFN-α, pegylated IFN-α, lamivudine, adefovir dipivoxil, entecavir, telbivudine, and tenofovir disoproxil fumarate.[1,3] Each agent has advantages and inherent limitations; pegylated IFN-α (given once a week) has the advantage of inducing a sustained virologic response after a defined course of treatment.[4–7] However, it has numerous side effects that limit its tolerability, a subcutaneous administration, and, importantly, is contraindicated in patients with decompensated HBV-related cirrhosis.

Nucleos(t)ide analogues (NAs) have the advantages of oral administration and favorable safety profiles with very potent antiviral effects. However, these drugs need to be administered continuously because withdrawal of therapy is generally associated with reactivation and a sustained response is uncommon except in HBeAg-positive patients who developed HBe seroconversion. In the case of HBe seroconversion, it is generally recommended to prolong therapy for at least 6 to 12 months before its withdrawal. The efficacy of lamivudine is limited by the emergence of lamivudine-resistant HBV. Adefovir is associated with a low incidence of resistance but its antiviral effect is not optimal. Entecavir, demonstrates an effectiveness against HBV and has a favorable safety profile with a low incidence of resistance. Telbivudine may have enhanced potency and lower rates of resistance than lamivudine but its resistance rate is significantly higher than other approved therapies. Tenofovir has been approved for chronic hepatitis B and several studies suggest that its resistance profile and its anti-HBV efficacy are superior to adefovir.

DECISION TO TREAT

The decision to treat patients with chronic HBV is primarily based on the severity of the liver disease. It is generally recommended to treat patients with chronic HBV with elevated alanine aminotransferase (ALT) levels and significant HBV replication. According to the European Association for the Study of the Liver clinical practice guidelines,[1] the indication to treat is based on the combination of the following 3 criteria: (1) serum HBV DNA levels, (2) serum ALT levels, and (3) histologic grade and stage of the liver disease. Patients should be considered for antiviral treatment when (1) serum HBV DNA is greater than 2000 IU/mL (ie, approximately 10,000 copies/mL), and/or (2) serum ALT levels are above the upper limit of normal, and (3) the liver biopsy specimen shows moderate to severe necroinflammation and/or fibrosis (eg, $\geq A2$ and/or $\geq F2$ if using the Metavir score). The fibrosis stage is the most important criteria to consider because it is the most important prognosis factor.

SUMMARY

If the decision is to treat with an analogy, we currently recommend de novo monotherapy with an agent that has a high genetic barrier to resistance, such as entecavir or tenofovir. With the highly potent, low-resistance drugs such as entecavir and tenofovir, the question of preventing resistance assumes far less importance. There is no evidence so far regarding the benefit of combination therapy with 2 analogues. Both entecavir and tenofovir have demonstrated considerable improvements in liver histology within long-term studies.

The progress made with new treatments has been important; however, further important goals of future research must be achieved: the eradication of covalently closed circular DNA (cccDNA), clarifying the role of serum HBsAg quantification in prediction of response,[18] new drugs and treatment strategies to improve seroconversion, as well as the prevention of HCC. Studies are ongoing on the potential superior efficacy of the combination of potent analogues with pegylated IFN.

REFERENCES

1. European Association for the Study of the Liver. EASL clinical practice guidelines: management of chronic hepatitis B virus infection. J Hepatol 2012;57: 167–85.
2. Chen CJ, Yang HI, Su J, et al. Risk of hepatocellular carcinoma across a biological gradient of serum hepatitis B virus DNA level. JAMA 2006;295:65–73.
3. Marcellin P, Asselah T, Boyer N. Treatment of chronic hepatitis B. J Viral Hepat 2005;12(4):333–45.
4. Lau GK, Piratvisuth T, Luo KX, et al. Peginterferon Alfa-2a, lamivudine, and the combination for HBeAg-positive chronic hepatitis B. N Engl J Med 2005; 352(26):2682–95.
5. Marcellin P, Lau GK, Bonino F, et al. Peginterferon alfa-2a alone, lamivudine alone, and the two in combination in patients with HBeAg-negative chronic hepatitis B. N Engl J Med 2004;351(12):1206–17.
6. Marcellin P, Bonino F, Lau GK, et al. Sustained response of hepatitis B e antigen-negative patients 3 years after treatment with peginterferon alpha-2a. Gastroenterology 2009;136(7):2169–79.
7. Buster EH, Hansen BE, Lau GK, et al. Factors that predict response of patients with hepatitis B e antigen positive chronic hepatitis B to peginterferon-alfa. Gastroenterology 2009;137:2002–9.
8. Marcellin P, Heathcote EJ, Buti M, et al. Tenofovir disoproxil fumarate versus adefovir dipivoxil for chronic hepatitis B. N Engl J Med 2008;359:2442–55.
9. Chang TT, Lai CL, Lim SG, et al. Entecavir treatment for up to 5 years in patients with hepatitis B e antigen-positive chronic hepatitis B. Hepatology 2010;51: 422–30.
10. Heathcote EJ, Marcellin P, Buti M, et al. Three year efficacy and safety of tenofovir disoproxil fumarate treatment for chronic hepatitis B. Gastroenterology 2011;140: 132–43.
11. Marcellin P, Heathcote EJ, Corsa A, et al. No detectable resistance to tenofovir disoproxil fumarate (TDF) following up to 240 weeks of treatment in patients with HBeAg+ and HBeAg- chronic hepatitis B virus infection. Hepatology 2011;54:480A.
12. Van Nunen AB, Hansen BE, Suh DJ, et al. Durability of HBeAg seroconversion following antiviral therapy for chronic hepatitis B: relation to type of therapy and

pre-treatment serum hepatitis B virus DNA and alanine aminotransferase. Gut 2003;53:420–4.

13. Lee HW, Lee HJ, Hwang JS, et al. Lamivudine maintenance beyond one year after HBeAg seroconversion is a major factor for sustained virologic response in HBeAg-positive chronic hepatitis B. Hepatology 2010;51:415–21.

14. Chang TT, Liaw YF, Wu SS, et al. Long-term entecavir therapy results in the reversal of fibrosis/cirrhosis and continued histological improvement in patients with chronic hepatitis B. Hepatology 2010;52:886–93.

15. Marcellin P, Gane E, Buti M, et al. Regression of cirrhosis during treatment with tenofovir disoproxil fumarate for chronic hepatitis B: a 5-year open-label follow-up study. Lancet 2013;381(9865):468–75.

16. Lampertico P, Vigano M, Soffredini R, et al. Entecavir monotherapy for nuc-naive chronic hepatitis B patients from field practice: high efficacy and favorable safety profile over 3 years. Hepatology 2011;54(Suppl 1) [Abstract 1436].

17. Lampertico P, Soffredini R, Vigano M, et al. 2-year effectiveness and safety of tenofovir in 302 NUC-naïve patients with chronic hepatitis B: a multicenter European study in clinical practice. Hepatology 2011;54(Suppl 1) [Abstract 1041A].

18. Martinot-Peignoux M, Lapalus M, Asselah T, et al. The role of HBsAg quantification for monitoring natural history and treatment outcome. Liver Int 2013;33(Suppl 1): 125–32.

Treatment of Patients with HBV-related Decompensated Cirrhosis and Liver Transplanted Patients

Bruno Roche, MD[a,b,c], Didier Samuel, MD, PhD[a,b,c],*

KEYWORDS

- Hepatitis B • Entecavir • Tenofovir • Cirrhosis • Liver transplantation
- Antiviral therapy • Hepatitis B immunoglobulin

KEY POINTS

- Antiviral therapy using newer nucleos(t)ide analogues with lower resistance rates such as entecavir or tenofovir could suppress HBV replication, improve liver function in patients with compensated or decompensated cirrhosis, delay or obviate the need for liver transplantation in some patients and reduce the risk of HBV recurrence.
- The combination of long-term antiviral and low-dose HBIG can effectively prevent HBV recurrence in >90% of transplant recipients. Some form of HBV prophylaxis needs be continued indefinitely post-transplant.
- In patients with a low-risk of HBV recurrence (i.e. HBV DNA levels undetectable pre-transplant) it is possible to discontinue HBIG and maintain long-term nucleos(t)ide analogue(s) therapy.
- A more cautious approach to prophylaxis regimen is necessary for those patients with high pre-transplant HBV DNA levels, those with limited antiviral options if HBV recurrence occur (ie, HIV or HDV coinfection, preexisting drug resistance), those with a high risk of HCC recurrence and those with a risk of non-compliance to antiviral therapy.
- Treatment of post-transplantation hepatitis B is a less important clinical problem than it was historically as effective antiviral therapies exist to rescue patients who failed initial prophylaxis.

INTRODUCTION

Approximately 15% to 30% of chronic hepatitis B virus (HBV) carriers are at increased risk of development of cirrhosis and complications of end-stage liver disease.[1] Antiviral therapy may stop viral replication and decrease the progression to cirrhosis,

The authors have nothing to disclose.

[a] AP-HP Hôpital Paul Brousse, Centre Hépato-Biliaire, Villejuif F-94800, France; [b] INSERM, Research Unit 785, Villejuif F-94800, France; [c] Univ Paris-Sud, Health Research Unit 785, Villejuif F-94800, France

* Corresponding author. Assistance Publique-Hopitaux de Paris, Hôpital Paul Brousse, Centre Hépato-Biliaire, 14 av P.V. Couturier, Villejuif 94804, France.

E-mail address: didier.samuel@pbr.aphp.fr

Clin Liver Dis 17 (2013) 451–473
http://dx.doi.org/10.1016/j.cld.2013.05.003
1089-3261/13/$ – see front matter © 2013 Elsevier Inc. All rights reserved.

liver.theclinics.com

hepatic decompensation, and hepatocellular carcinoma (HCC). During the last decade, the availability of new oral antiviral agents with a better safety profile, a higher efficacy, and a low rate of resistance development has significantly changed the management of end-stage liver disease caused by HBV. Nucleos(t)ides agents could suppress HBV replication and improve liver function in patients with compensated or decompensated cirrhosis[2–7] and delay or obviate liver transplantation (LT) in some patients.[8–10] Lamivudine (LAM) and adefovir (ADV) are no longer considered as an optimal first-line therapy related to a high rate of resistance development and latest guidelines suggest using entecavir (ETV) and tenofovir (TDV) as primary antiviral agents.[11,12] When LT is indicated for HCC or advanced liver failure, the use of nucleos(t)ides agents pretransplantation and the combination prophylaxis with nucleos(t)ides agents and hepatitis B immunoglobulin (HBIG) posttransplantation prevents HBV recurrence in 90% to 100% of patients and produces survival rates at 5 years of more than 80%. However, this long-term prophylaxis is expensive and inconvenient for patients. This has led to the development of alternative strategies to reduce the dose and duration of HBIG. Several effective drugs have been developed for the management of HBV disease on the graft so that outcome of recurrent HBV infection is currently good.

This article describes significant improvements in the management of end-stage liver disease caused by HBV over recent years and indications, results, and prevention of recurrence after LT for HBV-related liver disease.

NATURAL HISTORY OF HBV CIRRHOSIS

Liver cirrhosis is the end-stage in the natural history of chronic HBV infection. Several studies have evaluated the natural history of HBV cirrhosis. Approximately 20% of patients with compensated cirrhosis decompensate (ie, portal hypertension and variceal bleeding, ascites, jaundice, encephalopathy, liver failure, and HCC) over 5 years.[1] The study of de Jongh and colleagues[13] showed a marked decrease in survival among patients with decompensated cirrhosis and among patients positive for hepatitis B e antigen (HBeAg). They assessed survival of a cohort of 98 patients with HBV cirrhosis followed-up for a mean of 4.3 years. The 5-year survival rates were 72% and 97% for HBeAg-positive and HBeAg-negative patients with compensated cirrhosis and 0% and 28% for HBeAg-positive and HBeAg-negative patients with decompensated cirrhosis, respectively. Multivariate analysis showed that age, bilirubin, and ascites were independently related to survival. The risk of death was decreased by a factor of 2.2 when HBeAg seroconversion occurred during follow-up. Factors associated with an increased risk of liver failure include active viral replication, regular alcohol consumption, and coinfection with HIV or hepatitis C virus.[1,13] Another European multicenter longitudinal study was performed to assess the survival of hepatitis B surface antigen (HBsAg) positive compensated cirrhosis in 366 patients followed for a mean period of 72 months (6–202 months).[14] At entry 35% of the patients were HBeAg positive, 48% of the patients tested were HBV DNA positive by hybridization assay, and 20% anti–hepatitis delta virus (HDV) positive. Death occurred in 84 (23%) patients, mainly caused by liver failure (45 cases) or HCC (23 cases). The cumulative probability of survival was 84% and 68% at 5 and 10 years, respectively. Cox regression analysis identified six variables that independently correlated with survival: (1) age, (2) albumin, (3) platelets, (4) splenomegaly, (5) bilirubin, and (6) HBeAg positivity at time of diagnosis. Termination of HBV replication or biochemical remission during follow-up correlated with a highly significant better survival. These data show that in compensated cirrhosis, HBV replication, age, indirect indicators of poor hepatic reserve, and established portal hypertension significantly worsen the clinical course of the disease, whereas HDV infection does not influence the prognosis. The highly significant improvement in life expectancy after cessation of HBV replication favors antiviral therapy in these patients.

Risk factors for developing HCC in HBV-related cirrhosis include older age, male gender, severity of liver disease, active viral replication, viral genotype, viral mutants, hepatitis C virus or HDV-coinfection, alcohol intake, and aflatoxine exposure.[15] In studies conducted in East Asian countries and Europe or the United States, the cumulative 5-year incidences of HCC are 17% and 10%, respectively, in subjects with compensated cirrhosis.[1] The recommended regimen for HCC surveillance includes 6-monthly testing for α-fetoprotein and abdominal ultrasound. These patients should also be screened for varices and to assess the need for LT.

ANTIVIRAL THERAPY OF END-STAGE HBV LIVER DISEASE

The goals of treatment for patients with end-stage HBV liver disease are to improve liver function, thereby obviating LT, and in patients who require a transplant to decrease the risk of HBV recurrence posttransplant. The major factor to achieve these goals is to obtain sustained viral suppression and reduction in inflammatory hepatic activity. The approval of LAM was a major event in the treatment of HBV decompensated cirrhosis. The benefits of LAM therapy have been shown in several studies with a rapid viral suppression and an improvement of liver function (**Table 1**). However, the development of mutations in the HBV DNA polymerase gene is the main limitation of treatment with a reported incidence of 15% to 20% per year of therapy and a risk of fatal hepatitis flares.[2,3,9,16,17] ADV, a nucleotide analog, is an effective therapy for patients with wild-type and LAM-resistant HBV infection.[4] Although antiviral drug resistance is less common with ADV compared with LAM, concerns remain regarding the slow rate of suppressing HBV replication with ADV and the potential for dose-dependent nephrotoxicity in patients with decompensated HBV. LAM, telbivudine, and ADV are no longer considered as an optimal first-line therapy because of a high rate of resistance development or toxicity profile.

New nucleos(t)ides analogs, such as ETV and TDV, exhibit stronger antiviral efficacy and a lower resistance rate. They are recommended for the treatment of HBV infection in patients with end-stage liver disease; however, experience with these drugs is more limited in this setting.[11,12,18]

ETV, a nucleoside analog, is more potent in suppressing serum HBV DNA levels than LAM in HBeAg-positive and HBeAg-negative patients.[19,20] Because of a high genetic barrier of resistance this drug exhibits a very low resistance rate (ie, near 1%) in LAM-naive patients, even after 5 years of therapy.[21] In contrast, ETV resistance occurred in more than 35% of patients after 4 years of therapy in LAM-resistant patients.[22] In a recent study, Shim and colleagues[7] evaluated clinical outcome and virologic responses of 70 decompensated patients compared with 144 compensated patients treated with ETV (0.5 mg/day) as first-line therapy during 1 year (see **Table 1**). At Month 12 of therapy, the mean reduction in serum HBV DNA levels (-6.8 vs -6.7 $\log_{10}$ copies/mL), the proportion of patients achieving undetectable viremia (89% vs 78%) and the rate of HBeAg seroconversion (22% vs 24%) did not differ significantly between the decompensated and compensated groups. In the decompensated group, as reported with LAM, most adverse outcomes occurred within the first 6 months of therapy: six patients died because of liver failure and three patients underwent LT. These nine patients had more severe liver failure at entry compared with the other decompensated patients (Child-Pugh-Turcotte [CTP] score

Table 1
Results of antiviral therapy in patients with decompensated HBV-cirrhosis

Authors (Reference)	Antiviral Drug	Patients (% LAM-R)	Duration of Therapy (mo)	CTP Score at Entry	Decrease CTP ≥2 Pts (%)	HBV DNA Undetectable (%)	HBeAg Seroconversion (%)	LT (%)	Overall Survival (%)	Viral Breakthrough (%)
Villeneuve et al,[9] 2000	LAM	35	36	≥8	22/23 (96%)	23/23 (100%)	6/13 (46%)	7/35 (20%)	27/35 (77%)	2/23 (9%)
Perrillo et al,[3] 2001	LAM	77	38	NA	NA	17/22 (77%)	NA	NA	24/30 (80%)	3/18 (17%)
Fontana et al,[8] 2002	LAM	162	40	9	NA	57/71 (80%)	NA	91/162 (56%)	144/162 (89%)	18/162 (11%)
Hann et al,[17] 2003	LAM	75	13	≥7	23/75 (31%)	30/41 (73%)	7/36 (20%)	1/75 (1%)	64/75 (85%)	8/75 (11%)
Schiff et al,[4] 2007	ADV	226 (100%)	48	≥5	NA	45/76 (59%)	7/31 (23%)	43/226 (19%)	194/226 (86%)	2%
Shim et al,[7] 2010	ETV	70 (0)	12	≥7	27/55 (49%)	65/70 (93%)	8/35 (23%)	3/70 (4%)	63/70 (90%)	0
Liaw et al,[5] 2011	ADV	91 (33%)	24	≥7	25/91 (27%)	18/91 (20%)	5/51 (10%)	3/89 (3%)	73/89 (80%)	0 at wk 48 6 until wk 144
	ETV	100 (36%)	24	≥7	35/100 (35%)	57/100 (57%)	3/54 (6%)	11/100 (11%)	82/100 (82%)	0 at wk 48 3 until wk 144
Liaw et al,[6] 2011	ETV	22 (13%)	12	7–12	5/12 (42%)	16/22 (73%)	0/7 (0)	0/22 (0)	20/22 (91%)	0
	TDV	45 (18%)	12	7–12	7/27 (26%)	31/44 (71%)	3/14 (21%)	2/45 (4%)	43/45 (96%)	0
	TRU	45 (22%)	12	7–12	12/25 (48%)	36/41 (88%)	2/15 (13%)	4/45 (9%)	43/45 (96%)	0

Abbreviations: ADV, adefovir; CTP, Child-Pugh-Turcotte; ETV, entecavir; LAM, lamivudine; LT, liver transplantation; NA, not available; TDV, tenofovir; TRU, tenofovir + emtricitabine.

10.1 vs 8.1; P = .001); however, the baseline HBV DNA levels, the presence of HBeAg, and the early response to antiviral therapy were similar. Five patients developed HCC during the follow-up period. In a second study, 195 patients with decompensated HBV cirrhosis (positive or negative for HBeAg and experienced or naive for treatment with nucleos[t]ide analogs) were randomized to ETV (1 mg/day) or ADV (10 mg/day) (see **Table 1**).[5] The ETV group showed a greater change from baseline in HBV DNA at all time points through Week 48 and a higher proportion of subjects who achieved HBV DNA less than 300 copies/mL at Week 48 (ETV 57%; ADV 20%; $P<.0001$). Adverse events were comparable between groups. Safety of ETV in severely decompensated patients is poorly evaluated. A recent study showed that 5 of 16 patients with decompensated HBV-related disease (model for end-stage liver disease [MELD] score >20) developed symptomatic lactic acidosis leading to death in a patient with fulminant hepatitis B after receiving ETV for 4 to 240 days.[23] The mechanisms of toxicity are unclear; however, concomitant drugs, comorbidities, and other host factors may alter drug pharmacokinetic.

TDV, a nucleotide analog, is very potent against the wild-type and nucleosides analog-resistant HBV strains.[24] Phase III studies have shown that TDV has higher antiviral efficacy than ADV.[25] It has been shown that TDV can control HBV replication in most patients and can rescue LAM resistance or nonresponse to ADV. No drug-resistant variants have been reported with 5 years of continuous treatment.[25] TDV could be prescribed in combination with emtricitabine, a nucleoside analog with an antiviral activity profile similar to that of LAM (Truvada).

A recent study compared the safety and efficacy of TDV versus TDV plus emtricitabine versus ETV in 112 patients with decompensated HBV (see **Table 1**).[6] The frequency of undetectable HBV DNA at Weeks 12, 24, and 48 was comparable in the three treatment groups. However, among the subjects with LAM-resistant HBV, 71% of the 18 patients in the TDV-containing arms had undetectable HBV DNA at Week 48 compared with 33% in the three ETV-treated patients. Improvements in CTP and MELD scores at Week 48, rates of nephrotoxicity, and patient mortality were similar in the three treatment arms. There are growing concerns regarding the long-term safety of TDV in some patients including nephrotoxicity and metabolic bone disease.

Patients with decompensated cirrhosis should be treated in specialized liver units because the application of antiviral therapy is complex.[18] All studies emphasized the need for early treatment in patients with decompensated cirrhosis. Most studies have shown a biphasic survival pattern with most deaths occurring within the first 6 months of treatment.[4,7,8] Patients with higher pretreatment bilirubin levels, creatinin levels, and HBV DNA levels were at greatest risk for early death, whereas early suppression of HBV replication was not associated with more favorable outcomes.[7,8] Transplantation should not be delayed in patients with CTP class C or a MELD score greater than or equal to 15 at baseline, or be urgently considered in patients displaying suboptimal improvement in hepatic reserves after 3 months of antiviral treatment, because of the inability to identify those patients with a poor short-term prognosis (**Fig. 1**). Conversely, long-term antiviral treatment could be done in patients who can be stabilized with antiviral therapy.

The oral agents that most effectively suppress HBV replication with the lowest rate of drug resistance during prolonged use (ie, ETV, TDV) have emerged as preferred first-line agents over the other available drugs (LAM, ADV, telbivudine). Combination therapy using LAM and ADV could be used according to local health policies. Patients with decompensated HBV receiving oral nucleos(t)ides analogs must undergo frequent clinical and laboratory assessment to ensure medication compliance and

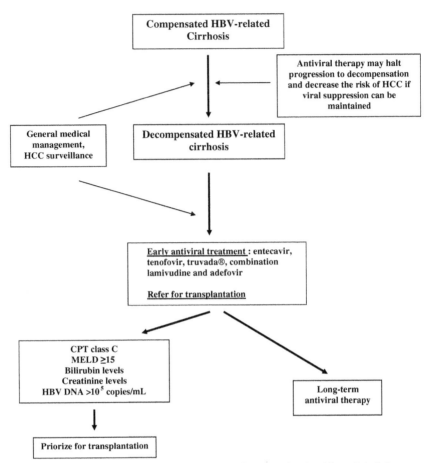

Fig. 1. Diagram of management of decompensated HBV cirrhosis with antiviral therapy and transplantation. CPT, Child-Pugh-Turcotte.

surveillance for virologic and clinical response and drug side effects, drug resistance, and HCC. Patients who fail to achieve primary response, as evidenced by a less than 2 $\log_{10}$ decrease in serum HBV DNA levels after 6 months of therapy, should be switched to an alternative treatment or receive additional treatment. Patients who develop breakthrough infection, defined by an increase of HBV DNA levels by more than 1 $\log_{10}$ from nadir, should be assessed for compliance to therapy and a test for antiviral-resistant mutation should be performed.

INDICATIONS AND RESULTS OF LT

In the United States and Europe, 5% to 10% of patients undergoing LT have HBV-associated liver disease.[10,26,27] In Asia, it is the most common indication for LT. When the expected median term survival is less than 2 years, LT should be considered. Transplantation is indicated in patients with a history of spontaneous bacterial peritonitis, chronic encephalopathy, refractory ascites, recurrent variceal bleeding despite endoscopic treatments, or HCC. Antiviral treatment using nucleos(t)ides analogs to suppress HBV replication may induce clinical improvement in a subset of patients and has led to a major decrease in the rate of LT for HBV cirrhosis. The main indications for LT in the setting of HBV cirrhosis are hepatitis flares related to viral resistance or noncompliance to antiviral therapy and HCC.[10,27] Kim and colleagues[10] report that several trends in the waiting list registration for LT for HBV-related disease in the United States have occurred, including an overall reduction in end-stage liver disease over time, along with persistent increase in HCC. In Europe, among patients transplanted for HBV-related disease, the proportion of patients transplanted for HCC increased from 15.8% in 1988 to 1995, to 29.6% in 2006 to 2010 (*P*<.001).[27] The impact of antiviral therapy on the incidence of HCC is less well established and delayed compared with that on end-stage liver disease. Wong and colleagues[28] report that despite more advanced liver disease and a lower rate of transplantation, intention-to-treat survival of patients listed for HBV cirrhosis is comparable with those with HBV cirrhosis and HCC, possibly related to beneficial effects of antiviral therapy.

Historically, in the absence of prophylaxis of HBV reinfection, the 5-year survival rate was low at between 40% and 60% and HBV-related deaths are frequent.[29,30] Major advances in prophylaxis and treatment of HBV recurrence have resulted in overall survival rates as high as 80% to 90% at 5 years.[26,27,31–33] In 206 European patients receiving adequate immunoprophylaxis, results of LT for HBV infection were similar to those results achieved with other indications, with survival rates at 1, 5, and 10 years of 91%, 81%, and 73%, respectively.[33] The 2-year patient survival increased from 85% in 1988 to 1993, to 94% after 1997 (*P*<.05) using prevention of HBV recurrence with HBIG and LAM. The 2-year recurrence rates in the two periods were 42% and 8% (*P*<.05). In the multivariate analysis for patient survival, only the covariates HCC and HBV recurrence were statistically significant. In our own series, the 10-year survival rate of patients who underwent LT for HBV cirrhosis and HDV cirrhosis was 70.9% and 89%, respectively.[34] A similar picture is seen in studies from the United States. The 5-year survival of HBV-infected transplant recipients has increased from 53% in the period 1987 to 1991 to 69% in the period 1992 to 1996, and to 76% in the period 1997 to 2002.[31]

DIAGNOSIS, MECHANISMS, AND RISK FACTORS FOR HBV RECURRENCE AFTER LT

Recurrence of HBV infection is commonly defined as the reappearance of circulating HBsAg and detectable HBV DNA after LT associated with an increase in transaminases levels and histologic evidence of acute or chronic hepatitis. However, measurable low levels of HBV DNA in serum, liver, and peripheral blood mononuclear cells or the presence of total and covalently closed circular HBV DNA in liver tissue could be detected transiently post-LT in the absence of a positive HBsAg, whatever the prophylaxis used.[34–38] The significance of these findings is unclear but suggests that occult HBV reinfection occurs in some HBV recipients after LT despite prophylaxis and implies a risk for overt HBV recurrence if the prophylaxis is stopped. In patients receiving antiviral monoprophylaxis, a persistence or reappearance of HBsAg positivity without detection of HBV DNA could be observed.[39,40] Some studies showed that part of the HBsAg production is independent from HBV DNA production.[41,42] The link between HBV DNA replication and HBsAg level is important but low production of HBsAg is coming from another pathway than HBV DNA replication explaining the low level of HBsAg observed in these patients. Control of viral replication involves interplay of HBV and immune responses, factors that are modified in the LT recipient by the use of antiviral prophylaxis and by immunosuppressive drugs. Conversely, for the few patients who are negative for HBV DNA and cccDNA in all compartments, the discontinuation of HBV prophylaxis could be discussed.[43] HBV reinfection could be the consequence of an immediate reinfection of the graft caused by circulating HBV particles; a later reinfection from HBV particles coming from extrahepatic sites, such as peripheral blood mononuclear cells; or both. In patients receiving HBIG, HBV reinfection may be the consequence of HBV overproduction coming from extrahepatic sites, an insufficient protective titer of anti–hepatitis B surface antibodies, or the emergence of escape mutant. This latter mechanism is probably important because mutations in the pre-S/S genome of HBV and in the "a" determinant have been described secondary to administration of HBIG.[44,45] Peripheral mononuclear cells may be implicated in this immune pressure selection mechanism; for example, we have shown that the HBV strain predominant in a patient after reinfection was the strain predominating in the mononuclear cells of this patient before LT.[46] This mechanism of escape mutation is not exclusive because HBV reinfection with a wild-type form of HBV occurs in patients receiving HBIG.[45] In patients receiving antiviral monoprophylaxis, such as LAM, HBsAg remained positive, progressively declining over a period of a few months after transplantation to become undetectable. When reinfection occurs in compliant patients treated with antiviral monotherapy, the emergence of mutations of the polymerase is the cause.[3] Reinfection in patients on HBIG and antivirals is related to combined mutations in the surface and polymerase genes.[47]

Whatever the prophylaxis used, the main risk factor of HBV recurrence is related to the pretransplant HBV viral load (ie, HBV DNA $>10^4$–10^5 copies/mL).[32,48–52] Earlier studies used hybridization assays that had a detection limit of approximately 10^5 copies/mL, whereas recent studies use more sensitive assays (polymerase chain reaction [PCR] or bDNA types), which have detection limits of approximately 10 copies/mL. Thus, the term "replicative HBV infection" has different meanings in different studies, depending on the HBV DNA test used. Other factors associated with low rates of recurrence are surrogate markers for low levels of viral replication and include negative HBeAg status at listing, fulminant HBV, and HDV coinfection.[32,50] Infection with LAM-resistant HBV virions (YMDD variants) increases the risk of recurrence regardless of viral load.[53,54] Several studies have recently reported that HCC at LT, HCC recurrence, or chemotherapy used for HCC is independently associated with an increased risk of HBV recurrence.[54–57]

POSTTRANSPLANT PREVENTION OF HBV RECURRENCE
Combination Prophylaxis

Since the study by Samuel and colleagues,[50] HBIG has been the cornerstone of prophylaxis against HBV recurrence post-LT. This study demonstrated a dramatic reduction in the rate of HBV recurrence, from 75% in patients receiving no or short-term therapy with HBIG, to 33% in those receiving long-term intravenous (IV) HBIG treatment ($P<.001$) and was associated with improved graft and patient survival. Recurrence of HBV occurred in 67% of patients who underwent transplantation for HBV cirrhosis, 32% of patients who underwent transplantation for HDV cirrhosis, and 17% of patients who underwent transplantation for fulminant hepatitis B. The HBV recurrence rate was related to the presence of HBV replication, which was assessed by HBeAg and HBV DNA detection in serum using conventional hybridization techniques at the time of LT. These results were confirmed by other clinical trials in the United States, Europe, and Asia and by long-term follow-up studies.[34,58–60] The advent of LAM further changed the landscape of post-LT prophylaxis and standard of care is now to combine HBIG with a nucleos(t)ide analog. Although its mechanism of action is incompletely understood, HBIG likely acts by binding to and neutralizing circulating virions and by inhibiting cell-to-cell infection.[61] HBIG had little effect on viral replication, as opposed to antivirals that directly inhibit HBV replication in hepatocytes and extrahepatic reservoirs. IV HBIG has been administered in two different ways: at a frequency dictated by the maintenance of specific anti-HBs levels (ie, 100 IU/L); or on a fixed schedule that generally "overshoots" the target anti-HBs level. The latter approach is simpler and requires less monitoring but is more expensive.[62] HBIG has a satisfactory safety record and adverse events observed have been usually minor. Evaluation of patients failing HBIG prophylaxis indicates that early recurrence of HBV post-LT is typically related to insufficient dosing of HBIG and is more frequent in patients with high level of pre-LT HBV replication, whereas late recurrences are usually caused by the emergence of mutations involving the "a" determinant of the HBV surface protein. The use of antivirals and HBIG post-LT provides complementary forms of prophylaxis posttransplantation to minimize risk of reinfection. Dickson and colleagues[63] reported that combination LAM and HBIG was associated with reduced requirements of HBs antibody to render the sera HBsAg negative early after LT. Combination prophylaxis allowed also a reduction of the dose of HBIG required in the long term. With this combination approach, the HBV recurrence rate at 1 to 2 years posttransplantation has been reduced to 0% to 10% (**Table 2**).[28,33,49,51,54–56,64–72] The use of IV HBIG has limitations, such as high cost, parenteral administration, limited supply, need for frequent clinic visits and laboratory monitoring, low effectiveness in patients with high levels of HBV replication before LT, and the potential selection of HBsAg escape mutants. To find less costly ways of providing HBIG prophylaxis long term, alternative approaches have been studied including the use of low-dose intramuscular (IM) HBIG,[64] subcutaneous HBIG,[73,74] withdrawal of HBIG after a finite period, or prophylaxis regimens without HBIG. The ability to achieve undetectable HBV DNA pre-LT in most patients using potent antivirals allows the use of prophylaxis regimens minimizing the dose or duration of HBIG.

Combination protocols are heterogeneous with regard to the dosing, duration, and routes of HBIG administration (see **Table 2**). The most cost-effective regimen reported to date is a very low IM HBIG plus LAM regimen.[64,68,75] Combination prophylaxis with low-dose IM HBIG (400–800 IU IM) decreased costs by more than 90% compared with IV regimen with a recurrence rate as low as 4% at 4 years.[64] Hooman and colleagues[75] report the result of a crossover study comparing IV with IM HBIG administration in stable liver recipients taking LAM or ADV more than 12 months after LT. They demonstrated comparability of elimination pharmacokinetics of HBIG regardless of the antibody route of administration, maintenance of protective anti-HBs levels, and no significant difference in the elimination characteristics as a function of pretransplant replication status. Taking efficacy and cost-effectiveness into consideration, IM HBIG plus LAM seems to be superior to IV HBIG plus LAM, although there may be a subset of patients (eg, high HBV DNA pretransplantation) who may benefit from the higher doses of HBIG provided by the IV route.[64] More recently, subcutaneous regimens of HBIG administered 6 months after LT have proved effective, with some advantage in tolerability and possibility of self-administration by patients at home.[73,74] Degertekin and colleagues[32] analyzed data from 183 patients who had undergone LT between 2001 and 2007. At transplant, 29% of patients were positive for HBeAg and 38.5% had high viral load (defined as HBV DNA >10^5 copies/mL). Posttransplant, all except six patients received combination prophylaxis with antiviral therapy (mostly LAM monotherapy) plus HBIG given either IV high dose (25%; 10,000 IU monthly); IV low dose (21.5%; 3000–6000 IU monthly); IM low dose (39%; 1000–1500 IU every 1–2 months); or for a finite duration (14.5%; median duration, 12 months). Cumulative rates of HBV recurrence at 1, 3, and 5 years were 3%, 7%, and 9%, respectively. Multivariate analysis showed that positivity for HBeAg and high viral load at transplant,

Table 2
Prevention of HBV recurrence after LT with antiviral and anti-HBs Ig (HBIG)

Authors (References)	No. of Patients	HBV DNA Positive at LT (%)	Prevention of HBV Recurrence	Follow-up (mo)	HBV Recurrence N (%)	Risk Factors for HBV Recurrence
Indefinite high-dose IV HBIG						
Markowitz et al,[69] 1998	14	1 (7%)	LAM + HBIG IV 10,000 IU/mo	13	0%	
Marzano et al,[65] 2001	25	0	LAM + HBIG IV 5000 IU/mo	30	4%	
Rosenau et al,[70] 2001	21	5 (23.8%)	LAM + HBIG IV titrated to maintain anti-HBs >200 U/L	20	9.5%	
Steinmuller et al,[33] 2002	206	NA	LAM or Famciclovir + HBIG IV titrated to maintain anti-HBs >100 U/L	NA	8%	
Faria et al,[55] 2008	51	21 (41%)	LAM ± ADV or TDV + HBIG IV 10,000 IU/mo	43	6.6%	HCC pre-LT Pre-LT HBV DNA $>10^5$ copies/mL HBIG monoprophylaxis
Han et al,[68] 2000	59	16 (27%)	LAM + HBIG IV 10,000 IU/mo	15	0%	NA
Chun et al,[54] 2010	186	76 (36.4%)	LAM + HBIG IV titrated to maintain anti-HBs >350 IU/L	35	10.2%	Recurrent HCC Pre-LT HBV DNA $>10^5$ copies/mL Lamivudine therapy for >1.5 y
Indefinite low-dose IM HBIG						
Gane et al,[64] 2007	147	125 (85%)	LAM + HBIG IM 400–800 IU/mo	17	1% 1 y 4% 5 y	Pre-LT HBV DNA
Zheng et al,[49] 2006	114	NA	LAM + HBIG IM 800 IU/mo	20	13.5% 1 y 15.2% 2 y	Pre-LT HBV DNA $>10^5$ copies/mL
Anselmo et al,[71] 2002	89	NA	LAM + HBIG IM 1560 IU/HBsAb level	29	11%	
Xi et al,[72] 2009	30 90	18 (60%) 52 (58%)	LAM + HBIG IM 800 IU/HBsAb level ETV + HBIG IM 800 IU/HBsAb level	NA	0% 11%	NA
Jiang et al,[66] 2010	254	53 (21%)	LAM + HBIG IM 800 IU/HBsAb level	41	2.3% 1 y 6.2% 3 y 8.2% 5 y	Pre-LT HBV DNA $>10^5$ copies/mL Prednisone withdrawal time >3 mo
Yi et al,[56] 2007	108	43 (40%)	LAM 1 y + HBIG IV 4000 IU/mo	31	13.8%	Cumulative dose corticoids Systemic therapy against HCC

Abbreviations: ADV, adefovir; ETV, entecavir; HCC, hepatocellular carcinoma; LAM, lamivudine; LT, liver transplantation; NA, not available; TDV, tenofovir.

but not the posttransplant HBIG regimen, were associated with HBV recurrence. Among the parameters of HBIG used that were evaluated in the systematic review of Cholongitas and colleagues,[76] only a high dosage during the first week after LT was found to be significantly associated with HBV recurrence.

Several meta-analyses have compared the use of HBIG, antivirals, or both.[76–79] Despite methodologic limitations of studies included in these meta-analyses, combination prophylaxis was significantly superior to antivirals or HBIG alone in preventing HBV recurrence, irrespective of the HBV DNA level at transplantation and reducing overall and HBV-related mortality in some studies. Cholongitas and colleagues[76] found that the combination of HBIG and ADV with or without LAM is more effective than the combination of HBIG and LAM for the prevention of HBV recurrence, which developed in 2% to 3% and 6% to 7% of patients, respectively (P<.05).

The optimal HBIG protocol is yet to be defined. Further research is needed to determine the dose and duration of HBIG after LT, appropriate titer levels of anti-HBs to prevent recurrence, and whether HBIG can be stopped. Most published studies used a combination of HBIG and LAM or ADV. The role and the safety of more potent nucleos(t)ide analogs (ETV or TDF) should be evaluated.[72,80]

Prophylaxis Protocols with Minimization of HBIG

Indefinite combination therapy with HBIG plus a nucleos(t)ide analog may not be required in all liver transplant recipients. The replication status of the patient before the initiation of antiviral therapy and at the time of LT should guide prophylaxis. Alternative strategies to consider, especially in patients without detectable HBV DNA before transplantation, are the discontinuation of HBIG after some defined interval and continuing treatment with antivirals alone, or adding HBsAg vaccination, or both. The high cost of long-term HBIG, the inconvenience of parenteral administration, and the use of potent antiviral agents prompt consideration of these other treatment approaches.

Studies of hepatitis B vaccination as an alternative to long-term HBIG in LT recipients were conducted in patients who were serum HBV DNA-negative before LT, with prolonged period of time from LT, who received low doses of immunosuppression, and were HBV DNA negative by PCR at the start of vaccination.[81–89] Anti-HBs titers achieved with the vaccination are highly variable and seem in part dependant of the type of vaccine: booster doses, double-dose third-generation recombinant vaccines, or addition of adjuvant. Patient populations and vaccine types, doses, schedules of administration, and definitions of response differed across these studies. From these data, it seems clear that successful hepatitis B vaccination and discontinuation of HBIG are feasible only in a small group of selected patients but the optimal vaccine protocol has not been established.

Two studies evaluated the efficacy of long-term HBIG monotherapy versus HBIG followed by LAM monotherapy in patients selected based on low risk of HBV reinfection.[90,91] At 1 year after the discontinuation of HBIG, the HBV reinfection rates were not significantly different; however, HBV DNA was detected by PCR in the serum of some patients without HBV recurrence. This latter finding suggests caution with this approach and the need for studies with longer follow-up and other antiviral therapy. Another strategy is HBIG withdrawal after a defined period of combination prophylaxis (**Table 3**).[28,43,67,92–96] In a study of 29 patients, high-dose HBIG and LAM were used in the first month, and then patients were randomized to receive either LAM monotherapy or LAM plus HBIG at 2000 IU IM monthly.[67] None of the patients developed HBV recurrence during the first 18 months but later recurrences developed in four patients after 5 years of follow-up related with poor LAM compliance.[92] Wong and colleagues[28]

Table 3
Prevention of HBV recurrence after LT with HBIG discontinuation and long-term antiviral therapy

Authors (References)	No. of Patients	HBV DNA Positive at LT (%)	Prevention of HBV Recurrence	Follow-up (mo)	HBV Recurrence N (%)
Buti et al,[67,92] 2007	29	0	Randomized trial LAM + HBIG 1 mo then LAM vs LAM + HBIG	83	1/15 (6.7%) in the LAM + HBIG group 3/14 (21.4%) in the LAM group (poor compliance to LAM)
Wong et al,[28] 2007	21	71%	HBIG ± LAM (median 26 mo) then LAM or ADV	40	1/21 (4.7%)
Neff et al,[95] 2007	10	0	LAM + HBIG 6 mo then LAM + ADV	31	0
Angus et al,[93] 2008	34	23%	Randomized trial Low-dose intramuscular HBIG + LAM >12 mo post-LT then HBIG + LAM vs ADV + LAM	21	0/18 in HBIG + LAM group 1/16 in ADV + LAM group
Saab et al,[94] 2011	61	22%	Intramuscular HBIG + LAM (>12 mo) then LAM or ETV + ADV or TDV	15	2/61 (3.3%)
Teperman et al,[96] 2011	37	47%	Randomized trial at a median of 3.4 y post-LT, HBIG + TDV-emtricitabine 24 wk then HBIG + TDV-emtricitabine vs TDV-emtricitabine	22	0

Abbreviations: ADV, adefovir; LAM, lamivudine; LT, liver transplantation; NA, not available; TDV, tenofovir.

reported HBV recurrence rates were 0% and 9% at 2 and 4 years after HBIG discontinuation. An alternative approach is to switch from HBIg/LAM to a combination of antiviral agents that present a greater barrier to the development of resistance than LAM. In a randomized prospective study, 16 of 34 patients receiving low-dose IM HBIG/LAM prophylaxis who were at least 12 months post-LT were switched to ADV/LAM combination therapy, whereas the remaining patients continued HBIG/LAM.[93] At a median follow-up of 21 months post-switch, no patient had disease recurrence, although one patient in the ADV/LAM group had a low titer of HBsAg in serum but was repeatedly HBV DNA negative. Using the same protocol, Saab and colleagues[94] switched 61 liver transplant recipients to a combination of a nucleoside (LAM or ETV) and nucleotide analog (ADV or TDV). At a median follow-up of 15 months postswitch, two patients were HBsAg positive in serum but repeatedly HBV DNA negative. Recently, Teperman and colleagues[96] evaluated the use of a combination of TDV with emtricitabine after HBIG discontinuation. In this study, subjects at a median of 3.4 years post-LT were treated with combination emtricitabine/TDV and HBIG for 24 weeks and then randomized to continue that prophylaxis regimen (N = 19) or discontinue HBIG (N = 18). At 72 weeks postrandomization, only one patient in the emtricitabine/TDV group had a transient detectability of HBV DNA related to poor compliance. Drug compliance during long-term antiviral therapy may be an important issue for transplant patients who feel healthy but have a lifelong risk of HBV recurrence. Safety data on the long-term use of ETV or TDV in transplant recipients are lacking. Consideration must be given to potential side effects: nephrotoxicity associated with TDV may be enhanced in transplant patients on calcineurin inhibitor therapy, risk of decreased bone density with TDV, and mitochondrial toxicity associated with ETV.

An ultimate approach was to evaluate the safety of complete and sustained prophylaxis withdrawal in liver transplant recipients at low risk of HBV recurrence. Lenci and colleagues,[43] evaluated a cohort of 30 patients at a low risk of recurrence (HBeAg and HBV DNA negative at LT, 23% HDV coinfected) and treated with combination HBIG and LAM (±ADV) for at least 3 years. Sequential liver biopsies were performed and evaluated for the presence of intrahepatic total HBV DNA and cccDNA. Using the absence of intrahepatic total HBV DNA and cccDNA as a guide, HBIG and then antiviral therapy was withdrawn in a stepwise fashion. After a median of 28.7 months off all prophylactic therapy, 83% of the cohort remained without serologic recurrence of HBV infection. Five patients developed HBsAg recurrence but only one patient showed evidence of HBV disease (HBV DNA positive); in the other patients HBsAg positivity was transient. Twenty-three of the 25 subjects without recurrence never had detectable HBV DNA in liver biopsies, whereas all five patients with recurrence had evidence of total HBV DNA in the liver and one had detected cccDNA. However, the ability to measure total HBV DNA and cccDNA in liver biopsy has limitations: this strategy needs sequential liver biopsies and assays for quantitation of total HBV DNA and cccDNA are not standardized.

The studies to date highlight several key issues to consider with the discontinuation of HBIG posttransplantation. First, the risk of HBV recurrence after cessation of HBIG may increase with time off HBIG either because of the development of viral resistance or because of nonadherence to antiviral therapy. The role of antivirals combination or antivirals with a high genetic barrier to resistance, such as ETV or TDV, should be evaluated. Second, the patients with high levels of HBV DNA at time of transplantation seem to be a higher-risk group for recurrence when HBIG is discontinued. Third, HBV DNA persists in serum, liver, or peripheral blood mononuclear cells even 10 years after LT in a proportion of HBV transplanted patients who are HBsAg-negative and these reservoirs may serve as a source of HBV reinfection in the future supporting the use of long-term prophylactic therapy in most patients.[34,35,38] Fourth, clinicians lack the ability to identify patients who may have cleared HBV posttransplantation.

HBIG-free Prophylactic Regimens

LAM has been evaluated as a prophylactic monotherapy, with the drug started pre-transplantation and continued posttransplantation without HBIG. The outcome at 1 year showed a 10% recurrence rate.[97] However, with longer follow-up, rates of recurrence reached 22% to 50% at 3 years post-LT (**Table 4**).[3,39,98,99] Recurrence was caused by the emergence of escape mutations in the YMDD motif of the polymerase gene and was observed mainly in patients with a high level of HBV replication before drug exposure. By reserving LAM monoprophylaxis for patients without viral replication at the time of LT, rates of recurrence can be lowered to less than 10%.[100] Because prophylactic therapy using LAM alone was associated with unacceptably high rates of reinfection in patients with a high level of viral replication before drug exposure, most transplant programs do not use LAM monotherapy for prophylaxis. Schiff and colleagues[4] reported 61 LAM-resistant patients treated with ADV in the wait-list who underwent LT. Sixty percent of these patients received post-LT HBIG and ADV combination prophylaxis and 40% ADV ± LAM prophylaxis. Interestingly, no patient in either group had recurrent HBV infection defined as two or more positive test results for HBsAg or for HBV DNA; however, follow-up was short (18 months). These studies showed the limitations of antiviral monoprophylaxis using LAM or ADV (see **Table 4**).[101] The emergence of drug resistance pre- or post-LT limits the efficacy of treatment. HBV DNA levels at the time of transplantation are related to pretreatment HBV DNA levels and duration of therapy and influence the risk of recurrence. The availability of more potent antivirals with a higher barrier to resistance could increase the proportion of patients with undetectable HBV DNA pretransplantation and decrease the risk of recurrent disease posttransplantation.[102] Wadhawan and colleagues[103] reported on 56 living donor recipients who received various antivirals pretransplant (LAM + ADV, N = 17; ETV, N = 25; TDV, N = 8; ETV + TDV, N = 2). Forty-seven out of 56 patients achieved an HBV DNA level lower than 2000 IU/mL before transplant and did not receive HBIG. All were HBV DNA undetectable after a median follow-up of 20 months posttransplant. Fung and colleagues[40] investigated the efficacy of ETV as monoprophylaxis in 80 patients with chronic hepatitis B who received a liver transplant. A total of 18 patients (22.5%) had persistent HBsAg positivity after transplant without seroclearance (N = 8) or reappearance of HBsAg after initial seroclearance (N = 10). Seventeen patients had undetectable levels of HBV DNA at the time of last follow-up. The remaining patient had a very low HBV DNA level of 217 copies/mL at 36 months post-LT. A key factor of HBsAg loss was the pretransplant quantitative HBsAg level. Whether other antivirals, such as TDV, or combination of antivirals without HBIG would provide effective prophylaxis is unknown.

Guidelines and Future Prospects for Prevention of HBV Reinfection

The principles in strategies to prevent HBV recurrence should be to maximize antiviral potency while minimizing the risk for viral resistance, costs, side effects, and inconvenience to patients. However, improvements in prophylactic regimens should not compromise the prevention of disease recurrence.

Viral suppression is the goal in every wait-listed patient. For those patients without viral replication pretransplant, there is no evidence that preoperative antiviral therapy is useful. For those patients with viral replication pretransplant, ETV, TDV, or a nucleoside/nucleotide combination should be used in preference to LAM or ADV.

Table 4
Prevention of HBV recurrence with antiviral monotherapy before and after LT

Authors (References)	No. of Patients	Patients HBV DNA Positive at Time of Treatment	Patients HBeAg Positive at Time of Treatment	Duration of Treatment Before LT	Patients HBV DNA Positive at Time of LT	No. of LT	No. of HBV Recurrence (%)	Follow-up (mo)	Death Related to HBV Recurrence
Lamivudine									
Grellier et al,[97] 1996; Mutimer et al,[99] 2000	17	8	4	2 (1.2–5.6)	0	12	5 (50%)	32 (16–51)	2
Lo et al,[39] 2001	31	11	18	1.6 (0.03–20.4)	6	31	7[a] (22.6%)	16 (6–47)	0
Perillo et al,[3] 2001	77	26	24	2.1 (0.03–20.9)	6	47	17 (36.1%)	38 (2.7–48.5)	1
Zheng et al,[49] 2006	51	51	NA	0	51	51	21 (41.1%)	29.8 (6.5–60)	3
Lamivudine + Adefovir									
Lo et al,[101] 2005	8	8	NA	LAM 30 (16.8–59.9) ADV 2.9 (0–9)	7	8	2[b] (25%)	11.5 (4.4–26)	0
Schiff et al,[4] 2007	23	23	NA	LAM (NA) ADV 5 (NA)	NA	23	3[c] (13%)	9 (NA)	0
Entecavir									
Fung et al,[40] 2011	80	NA	NA	5 (0–44) 47 treated patients (LAM, ADV, ETV)	59	80	18[d] (22.5%)	26 (5–40)	0

Abbreviations: HBeAg, hepatitis B e antigen; HBV, hepatitis B virus; LT, orthotopic liver transplantation; NA, not available; PCR, polymerase chain reaction.
[a] Six of these patients were HBsAg positive, HBV DNA negative by PCR.
[b] These two patients were HBsAg positive, HBV DNA negative by PCR.
[c] Two of these patients were HBsAg positive and 3 HBV DNA positive.
[d] Seventeen of these patients were HBsAg positive, HBV DNA negative by PCR.

There is a consensus regarding the need for a life-long prophylactic therapy supported by the detection of HBV DNA in hepatic and extrahepatic sites in patients who are HBsAg negative on posttransplant HBIG and antivirals. Today, low-dose IM HBIg in combination with a potent nucleos(t)ide analog is the most cost-effective prophylaxis. Patients with undetectable HBV DNA levels at the time of transplant are eligible for protocols using short-term low-dose IM HBIG and antiviral then switched to antiviral monotherapy or combination therapy (**Fig. 2**). A more cautious approach to prophylaxis regimen is necessary for those patients with high pretransplant HBV DNA levels; those with limited antiviral options if HBV recurrence occurred (ie, HIV or HDV coinfection, preexisting drug resistance or intolerance); those with a high risk of HCC recurrence; and those with a risk of noncompliance to antiviral therapy. In this group, HBIG-free prophylaxis cannot be recommended.

HBV RECURRENCE

Most cases of HBV reinfection occur during the first 3 years after transplantation and rarely thereafter.[34] HBV reinfection is characterized by the appearance of HBsAg in serum. The HBV replication level is usually high, and large amounts of HBV particles are present in the graft. Historically, before the advent of antivirals, HBV reinfection had a major impact on graft and patient survival because almost all patients with HBV reinfection developed graft disease.[29,30] In most cases, acute lobular hepatitis occurred with an evolution to chronic active hepatitis. In some cases, acute liver failure was observed. This severe evolution was probably related to the high amount of HBsAg, HBeAg, and hepatitis B core antigen present in the nuclei and the cytoplasm of the hepatocytes, suggesting that liver injury is caused by a direct cytopathic effect of the virus. A particular form of virus recurrence was called "fibrosing cholestatic hepatitis." Antiviral treatments have dramatically improved the prognosis of HBV graft

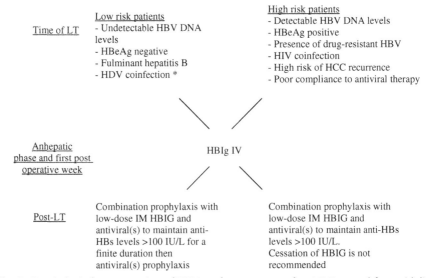

Fig. 2. Prophylaxis for prevention of HBV graft recurrence after LT. Proposal for guideline. * Shortening the duration of HBIG administration in patients with HDV/HBV could have detrimental consequences because reinfection in the case of HDV latency may lead to chronic hepatitis B and delta.

reinfection. The treatment of HBV infection is mandatory because of the severity of the liver graft disease in relation to a high viral load. HBV infection after LT is usually the result of failed prophylaxis, either because of noncompliance or the development of drug-resistant HBV infection. The availability of safe and effective antivirals allows most patients with recurrent infection to survive without graft loss from recurrent disease. Selection of therapy for HBV infection depends on treatments previously received by patients (ie, no therapy, HBIG alone, antiviral alone, or HBIG and antiviral in combination). The optimal management strategy to ensure long-term HBV suppression is predicted to be the use of an antiviral with high genetic barrier to the development of resistance, such as ETV or TDV, or the use of combinations of antivirals. A close monitoring for initial response and for subsequent virologic breakthrough is essential to prevent disease progression and flares of hepatitis. Patients with a suboptimal response warrant a change of therapy. In patients who are naive to treatment or with S gene mutants, ETV or TDV is the drug of choice as single agents but combination therapy could be considered. LAM or ADV is not recommended as a single agent because of a high risk of resistance. In those patients with LAM-resistant HBV, ADV or TDV in combination with LAM has been shown to be effective.[4,104] In those patients with ADV-resistant HBV, LAM or ETV in combination with ADV has been shown to be effective.[105] In summary, long-term suppression of HBV replication is essential to prevent disease progression, prior drug exposure and achieved resistances mutations are important in guiding drug choices, and combination antiviral therapy is recommended over sequential antiviral use to minimize the risk of treatment failure.

SUMMARY

During the past two decades, major advances have been made in the management of HBV transplant candidates. The advent of long-term HBIG administration and efficient antiviral drugs used pretransplant and posttransplant as a prophylaxis of HBV recurrence were major breakthroughs in the management of patients. The combination of long-term antiviral and low-dose HBIG can effectively prevent HBV recurrence in more than 90% of transplant recipients. Some form of HBV prophylaxis needs be continued indefinitely posttransplant. However, in patients with low HBV DNA levels pretransplantation, discontinuation of HBIG with continued long-term nucleos(t)ide analog(s) treatment is possible.

Currently, treatment of posttransplantation hepatitis B is a less important clinical problem than it was historically. Effective antiviral therapies exist to rescue patients who failed initial prophylaxis. New HBV antivirals, such as ETV and TDV, are effective in viral suppression of resistant variants.

REFERENCES

1. Fattovich G, Bortolotti F, Donato F. Natural history of chronic hepatitis B: special emphasis on disease progression and prognostic factors. J Hepatol 2008;48(2): 335–52.
2. Yao FY, Terrault NA, Freise C, et al. Lamivudine treatment is beneficial in patients with severely decompensated cirrhosis and actively replicating hepatitis B infection awaiting liver transplantation: a comparative study using a matched, untreated cohort. Hepatology 2001;34(2):411–6.
3. Perrillo RP, Wright T, Rakela J, et al. A multicenter United States-Canadian trial to assess lamivudine monotherapy before and after liver transplantation for chronic hepatitis B. Hepatology 2001;33(2):424–32.

4. Schiff E, Lai CL, Hadziyannis S, et al. Adefovir dipivoxil for wait-listed and post-liver transplantation patients with lamivudine-resistant hepatitis B: final long-term results. Liver Transpl 2007;13(3):349–60.

5. Liaw YF, Raptopoulou-Gigi M, Cheinquer H, et al. Efficacy and safety of entecavir versus adefovir in chronic hepatitis B patients with hepatic decompensation: a randomized, open-label study. Hepatology 2011;54(1):91–100.

6. Liaw YF, Sheen IS, Lee CM, et al. Tenofovir disoproxil fumarate (TDF), emtricitabine/TDF, and entecavir in patients with decompensated chronic hepatitis B liver disease. Hepatology 2011;53(1):62–72.

7. Shim JH, Lee HC, Kim KM, et al. Efficacy of entecavir in treatment-naive patients with hepatitis B virus-related decompensated cirrhosis. J Hepatol 2010;52(2): 176–82.

8. Fontana RJ, Hann HW, Perrillo RP, et al. Determinants of early mortality in patients with decompensated chronic hepatitis B treated with antiviral therapy. Gastroenterology 2002;123(3):719–27.

9. Villeneuve JP, Condreay LD, Willems B, et al. Lamivudine treatment for decompensated cirrhosis resulting from chronic hepatitis B. Hepatology 2000;31(1): 207–10.

10. Kim WR, Terrault NA, Pedersen RA, et al. Trends in waiting list registration for liver transplantation for viral hepatitis in the United States. Gastroenterology 2009;137(5):1680–6.

11. European Association For The Study Of The Liver. EASL clinical practice guidelines: management of chronic hepatitis B. J Hepatol 2009;50(2):227–42.

12. Lok AS, McMahon BJ. Chronic hepatitis B: update 2009. Hepatology 2009; 50(3):661–2.

13. de Jongh FE, Janssen HL, de Man RA, et al. Survival and prognostic indicators in hepatitis B surface antigen-positive cirrhosis of the liver. Gastroenterology 1992;103(5):1630–5.

14. Realdi G, Fattovich G, Hadziyannis S, et al. Survival and prognostic factors in 366 patients with compensated cirrhosis type B: a multicenter study. The Investigators of the European Concerted Action on Viral Hepatitis (EUROHEP). J Hepatol 1994;21(4):656–66.

15. Fattovich G, Stroffolini T, Zagni I, et al. Hepatocellular carcinoma in cirrhosis: incidence and risk factors. Gastroenterology 2004;127(5 Suppl 1):S35–50.

16. Fontana RJ, Keeffe EB, Carey W, et al. Effect of lamivudine treatment on survival of 309 North American patients awaiting liver transplantation for chronic hepatitis B. Liver Transpl 2002;8(5):433–9.

17. Hann HW, Fontana RJ, Wright T, et al. A United States compassionate use study of lamivudine treatment in nontransplantation candidates with decompensated hepatitis B virus-related cirrhosis. Liver Transpl 2003;9(1):49–56.

18. Singal AK, Fontana RJ. Meta-analysis: oral anti-viral agents in adults with decompensated hepatitis B virus cirrhosis. Aliment Pharmacol Ther 2012;35(6): 674–89.

19. Chang TT, Gish RG, de Man R, et al. A comparison of entecavir and lamivudine for HBeAg-positive chronic hepatitis B. N Engl J Med 2006;354(10): 1001–10.

20. Lai CL, Shouval D, Lok AS, et al. Entecavir versus lamivudine for patients with HBeAg-negative chronic hepatitis B. N Engl J Med 2006;354(10):1011–20.

21. Tenney DJ, Rose RE, Baldick CJ, et al. Long-term monitoring shows hepatitis B virus resistance to entecavir in nucleoside-naive patients is rare through 5 years of therapy. Hepatology 2009;49(5):1503–14.

22. Sherman M, Yurdaydin C, Sollano J, et al. Entecavir for treatment of lamivudine-refractory, HBeAg-positive chronic hepatitis B. Gastroenterology 2006;130(7): 2039–49.

23. Lange CM, Bojunga J, Hofmann WP, et al. Severe lactic acidosis during treatment of chronic hepatitis B with entecavir in patients with impaired liver function. Hepatology 2009;50(6):2001–6.

24. van Bommel F, Zollner B, Sarrazin C, et al. Tenofovir for patients with lamivudine-resistant hepatitis B virus (HBV) infection and high HBV DNA level during adefovir therapy. Hepatology 2006;44(2):318–25.

25. Marcellin P, Heathcote EJ, Buti M, et al. Tenofovir disoproxil fumarate versus adefovir dipivoxil for chronic hepatitis B. N Engl J Med 2008;359(23):2442–55.

26. European Liver Transplant Registry. Available at: http://www.eltr.org. Accessed June 17, 2013.

27. Burra P, Germani G, Adam R, et al. Liver transplantation for HBV-related cirrhosis in Europe: a ELTR study on evolution and outcomes. J Hepatol 2013; 58(2):287–96.

28. Wong SN, Chu CJ, Wai CT, et al. Low risk of hepatitis B virus recurrence after withdrawal of long-term hepatitis B immunoglobulin in patients receiving maintenance nucleos(t)ide analogue therapy. Liver Transpl 2007;13(3):374–81.

29. Todo S, Demetris AJ, Van Thiel D, et al. Orthotopic liver transplantation for patients with hepatitis B virus-related liver disease. Hepatology 1991;13(4): 619–26.

30. O'Grady JG, Smith HM, Davies SE, et al. Hepatitis B virus reinfection after orthotopic liver transplantation. Serological and clinical implications. J Hepatol 1992; 14(1):104–11.

31. Kim WR, Poterucha JJ, Kremers WK, et al. Outcome of liver transplantation for hepatitis B in the United States. Liver Transpl 2004;10(8):968–74.

32. Degertekin B, Han SH, Keeffe EB, et al. Impact of virologic breakthrough and HBIG regimen on hepatitis B recurrence after liver transplantation. Am J Transplant 2010;10(8):1823–33.

33. Steinmuller T, Seehofer D, Rayes N, et al. Increasing applicability of liver transplantation for patients with hepatitis B-related liver disease. Hepatology 2002; 35(6):1528–35.

34. Roche B, Feray C, Gigou M, et al. HBV DNA persistence 10 years after liver transplantation despite successful anti-HBS passive immunoprophylaxis. Hepatology 2003;38(1):86–95.

35. Hussain M, Soldevila-Pico C, Emre S, et al. Presence of intrahepatic (total and ccc) HBV DNA is not predictive of HBV recurrence after liver transplantation. Liver Transpl 2007;13(8):1137–44.

36. Freshwater DA, Dudley T, Cane P, et al. Viral persistence after liver transplantation for hepatitis B virus: a cross-sectional study. Transplantation 2008;85(8): 1105–11.

37. Yasunaka T, Takaki A, Yagi T, et al. Serum hepatitis B virus DNA before liver transplantation correlates with HBV reinfection rate even under successful low-dose hepatitis B immunoglobulin prophylaxis. Hepatol Int 2011;5(4):918–26.

38. Coffin CS, Mulrooney-Cousins PM, van Marle G, et al. Hepatitis B virus quasispecies in hepatic and extrahepatic viral reservoirs in liver transplant recipients on prophylactic therapy. Liver Transpl 2011;17(8):955–62.

39. Lo CM, Cheung ST, Lai CL, et al. Liver transplantation in Asian patients with chronic hepatitis B using lamivudine prophylaxis. Ann Surg 2001;233(2): 276–81.

40. Fung J, Cheung C, Chan SC, et al. Entecavir monotherapy is effective in suppressing hepatitis B virus after liver transplantation. Gastroenterology 2011; 141(4):1212–9.

41. Brunetto MR. A new role for an old marker, HBsAg. J Hepatol 2010;52(4):475–7.

42. Nguyen T, Thompson AJ, Bowden S, et al. Hepatitis B surface antigen levels during the natural history of chronic hepatitis B: a perspective on Asia. J Hepatol 2010;52(4):508–13.

43. Lenci I, Tisone G, Di Paolo D, et al. Safety of complete and sustained prophylaxis withdrawal in patients liver-transplanted for HBV-related cirrhosis at low risk of HBV recurrence. J Hepatol 2011;55(3):587–93.

44. Ghany MG, Ayola B, Villamil FG, et al. Hepatitis B virus S mutants in liver transplant recipients who were reinfected despite hepatitis B immune globulin prophylaxis. Hepatology 1998;27(1):213–22.

45. Terrault NA, Zhou S, McCory RW, et al. Incidence and clinical consequences of surface and polymerase gene mutations in liver transplant recipients on hepatitis B immunoglobulin. Hepatology 1998;28(2):555–61.

46. Brind A, Jiang J, Samuel D, et al. Evidence for selection of hepatitis B mutants after liver transplantation through peripheral blood mononuclear cell infection. J Hepatol 1997;26(2):228–35.

47. Bock CT, Tillmann HL, Torresi J, et al. Selection of hepatitis B virus polymerase mutants with enhanced replication by lamivudine treatment after liver transplantation. Gastroenterology 2002;122(2):264–73.

48. Marzano A, Gaia S, Ghisetti V, et al. Viral load at the time of liver transplantation and risk of hepatitis B virus recurrence. Liver Transpl 2005;11(4):402–9.

49. Zheng S, Chen Y, Liang T, et al. Prevention of hepatitis B recurrence after liver transplantation using lamivudine or lamivudine combined with hepatitis B Immunoglobulin prophylaxis. Liver Transpl 2006;12(2):253–8.

50. Samuel D, Muller R, Alexander G, et al. Liver transplantation in European patients with the hepatitis B surface antigen. N Engl J Med 1993;329(25):1842–7.

51. Neff GW, O'Brien CB, Nery J, et al. Outcomes in liver transplant recipients with hepatitis B virus: resistance and recurrence patterns from a large transplant center over the last decade. Liver Transpl 2004;10(11):1372–8.

52. Mutimer D, Pillay D, Dragon E, et al. High pre-treatment serum hepatitis B virus titre predicts failure of lamivudine prophylaxis and graft re-infection after liver transplantation. J Hepatol 1999;30(4):715–21.

53. Xie SB, Zhu JY, Ying Z, et al. Prevention and risk factors of the HBV recurrence after orthotopic liver transplantation: 160 cases follow-up study. Transplantation 2010;90(7):786–90.

54. Chun J, Kim W, Kim BG, et al. High viremia, prolonged lamivudine therapy and recurrent hepatocellular carcinoma predict posttransplant hepatitis B recurrence. Am J Transplant 2010;10(7):1649–59.

55. Faria LC, Gigou M, Roque-Afonso AM, et al. Hepatocellular carcinoma is associated with an increased risk of hepatitis B virus recurrence after liver transplantation. Gastroenterology 2008;134(7):1890–9 [quiz: 2155].

56. Yi NJ, Suh KS, Cho JY, et al. Recurrence of hepatitis B is associated with cumulative corticosteroid dose and chemotherapy against hepatocellular carcinoma recurrence after liver transplantation. Liver Transpl 2007;13(3):451–8.

57. Saab S, Yeganeh M, Nguyen K, et al. Recurrence of hepatocellular carcinoma and hepatitis B reinfection in hepatitis B surface antigen-positive patients after liver transplantation. Liver Transpl 2009;15(11):1525–34.

58. Terrault NA, Zhou S, Combs C, et al. Prophylaxis in liver transplant recipients using a fixed dosing schedule of hepatitis B immunoglobulin. Hepatology 1996; 24(6):1327–33.
59. Muller R, Gubernatis G, Farle M, et al. Liver transplantation in HBs antigen (HBsAg) carriers. Prevention of hepatitis B virus (HBV) recurrence by passive immunization. J Hepatol 1991;13(1):90–6.
60. Hwang S, Ahn CS, Song GW, et al. Posttransplantation prophylaxis with primary high-dose hepatitis B immunoglobulin monotherapy and complementary preemptive antiviral add-on. Liver Transpl 2011;17(4):456–65.
61. Shouval D, Samuel D. Hepatitis B immune globulin to prevent hepatitis B virus graft reinfection following liver transplantation: a concise review. Hepatology 2000;32(6):1189–95.
62. Di Paolo D, Tisone G, Piccolo P, et al. Low-dose hepatitis B immunoglobulin given "on demand" in combination with lamivudine: a highly cost-effective approach to prevent recurrent hepatitis B virus infection in the long-term follow-up after liver transplantation. Transplantation 2004;77(8):1203–8.
63. Dickson RC, Terrault NA, Ishitani M, et al. Protective antibody levels and dose requirements for IV 5% Nabi hepatitis B immune globulin combined with lamivudine in liver transplantation for hepatitis B-induced end stage liver disease. Liver Transpl 2006;12(1):124–33.
64. Gane EJ, Angus PW, Strasser S, et al. Lamivudine plus low-dose hepatitis B immunoglobulin to prevent recurrent hepatitis B following liver transplantation. Gastroenterology 2007;132(3):931–7.
65. Marzano A, Salizzoni M, Debernardi-Venon W, et al. Prevention of hepatitis B virus recurrence after liver transplantation in cirrhotic patients treated with lamivudine and passive immunoprophylaxis. J Hepatol 2001;34(6):903–10.
66. Jiang L, Yan L, Li B, et al. Prophylaxis against hepatitis B recurrence posttransplantation using lamivudine and individualized low-dose hepatitis B immunoglobulin. Am J Transplant 2010;10(8):1861–9.
67. Buti M, Mas A, Prieto M, et al. A randomized study comparing lamivudine monotherapy after a short course of hepatitis B immune globulin (HBIg) and lamivudine with long-term lamivudine plus HBIg in the prevention of hepatitis B virus recurrence after liver transplantation. J Hepatol 2003;38(6): 811–7.
68. Han SH, Ofman J, Holt C, et al. An efficacy and cost-effectiveness analysis of combination hepatitis B immune globulin and lamivudine to prevent recurrent hepatitis B after orthotopic liver transplantation compared with hepatitis B immune globulin monotherapy. Liver Transpl 2000;6(6):741–8.
69. Markowitz JS, Martin P, Conrad AJ, et al. Prophylaxis against hepatitis B recurrence following liver transplantation using combination lamivudine and hepatitis B immune globulin. Hepatology 1998;28(2):585–9.
70. Rosenau J, Bahr MJ, Tillmann HL, et al. Lamivudine and low-dose hepatitis B immune globulin for prophylaxis of hepatitis B reinfection after liver transplantation possible role of mutations in the YMDD motif prior to transplantation as a risk factor for reinfection. J Hepatol 2001;34(6):895–902.
71. Anselmo DM, Ghobrial RM, Jung LC, et al. New era of liver transplantation for hepatitis B: a 17-year single-center experience. Ann Surg 2002;235(5):611–9 [discussion: 619–20].
72. Xi ZF, Xia Q, Zhang JJ, et al. The role of entecavir in preventing hepatitis B recurrence after liver transplantation. J Dig Dis 2009;10(4):321–7.

73. Singham J, Greanya ED, Lau K, et al. Efficacy of maintenance subcutaneous hepatitis B immune globulin (HBIG) post-transplant for prophylaxis against hepatitis B recurrence. Ann Hepatol 2011;9(2):166–71.

74. Yahyazadeh A, Beckebaum S, Cicinnati V, et al. Efficacy and safety of subcutaneous human HBV-immunoglobulin (Zutectra) in liver transplantation: an open, prospective, single-arm phase III study. Transpl Int 2011;24(5):441–50.

75. Hooman N, Rifai K, Hadem J, et al. Antibody to hepatitis B surface antigen trough levels and half-lives do not differ after intravenous and intramuscular hepatitis B immunoglobulin administration after liver transplantation. Liver Transpl 2008;14(4):435–42.

76. Cholongitas E, Goulis J, Akriviadis E, et al. Hepatitis B immunoglobulin and/or nucleos(t)ide analogues for prophylaxis against hepatitis b virus recurrence after liver transplantation: a systematic review. Liver Transpl 2011;17(10): 1176–90.

77. Rao W, Wu X, Xiu D. Lamivudine or lamivudine combined with hepatitis B immunoglobulin in prophylaxis of hepatitis B recurrence after liver transplantation: a meta-analysis. Transpl Int 2009;22(4):387–94.

78. Katz LH, Paul M, Guy DG, et al. Prevention of recurrent hepatitis B virus infection after liver transplantation: hepatitis B immunoglobulin, antiviral drugs, or both? Systematic review and meta-analysis. Transpl Infect Dis 2009;12(4):292–308.

79. Loomba R, Rowley AK, Wesley R, et al. Hepatitis B immunoglobulin and lamivudine improve hepatitis B-related outcomes after liver transplantation: meta-analysis. Clin Gastroenterol Hepatol 2008;6(6):696–700.

80. Jimenez-Perez M, Saez-Gomez AB, Mongil Poce L, et al. Efficacy and safety of entecavir and/or tenofovir for prophylaxis and treatment of hepatitis B recurrence post-liver transplant. Transplant Proc 2010;42(8):3167–8.

81. Sanchez-Fueyo A, Rimola A, Grande L, et al. Hepatitis B immunoglobulin discontinuation followed by hepatitis B virus vaccination: a new strategy in the prophylaxis of hepatitis B virus recurrence after liver transplantation. Hepatology 2000;31(2):496–501.

82. Angelico M, Di Paolo D, Trinito MO, et al. Failure of a reinforced triple course of hepatitis B vaccination in patients transplanted for HBV-related cirrhosis. Hepatology 2002;35(1):176–81.

83. Bienzle U, Gunther M, Neuhaus R, et al. Immunization with an adjuvant hepatitis B vaccine after liver transplantation for hepatitis B-related disease. Hepatology 2003;38(4):811–9.

84. Albeniz Arbizu E, Barcena Marugan R, Oton Nieto E, et al. Prophylaxis of recurrent hepatitis B virus by vaccination after liver transplant: preliminary results. Transplant Proc 2003;35(5):1848–9.

85. Lo CM, Liu CL, Chan SC, et al. Failure of hepatitis B vaccination in patients receiving lamivudine prophylaxis after liver transplantation for chronic hepatitis B. J Hepatol 2005;43(2):283–7.

86. Rosenau J, Hooman N, Hadem J, et al. Failure of hepatitis B vaccination with conventional HBsAg vaccine in patients with continuous HBIG prophylaxis after liver transplantation. Liver Transpl 2007;13(3):367–73.

87. Weber NK, Forman LM, Trotter JF. HBIg discontinuation with maintenance oral anti-viral therapy and HBV vaccination in liver transplant recipients. Dig Dis Sci 2010;55(2):505–9.

88. Di Paolo D, Lenci I, Cerocchi C, et al. One-year vaccination against hepatitis B virus with a MPL-vaccine in liver transplant patients for HBV-related cirrhosis. Transpl Int 2010;23(11):1105–12.

89. Gunther M, Neuhaus R, Bauer T, et al. Immunization with an adjuvant hepatitis B vaccine in liver transplant recipients: antibody decline and booster vaccination with conventional vaccine. Liver Transpl 2006;12(2):316–9.

90. Dodson SF, de Vera ME, Bonham CA, et al. Lamivudine after hepatitis B immune globulin is effective in preventing hepatitis B recurrence after liver transplantation. Liver Transpl 2000;6(4):434–9.

91. Naoumov NV, Lopes AR, Burra P, et al. Randomized trial of lamivudine versus hepatitis B immunoglobulin for long-term prophylaxis of hepatitis B recurrence after liver transplantation. J Hepatol 2001;34(6):888–94.

92. Buti M, Mas A, Prieto M, et al. Adherence to lamivudine after an early withdrawal of hepatitis B immune globulin plays an important role in the long-term prevention of hepatitis B virus recurrence. Transplantation 2007;84(5):650–4.

93. Angus PW, Patterson SJ, Strasser SI, et al. A randomized study of adefovir dipivoxil in place of HBIG in combination with lamivudine as post-liver transplantation hepatitis B prophylaxis. Hepatology 2008;48(5):1460–6.

94. Saab S, Desai S, Tsaoi D, et al. Posttransplantation hepatitis B prophylaxis with combination oral nucleoside and nucleotide analog therapy. Am J Transplant 2011;11(3):511–7.

95. Neff GW, Kemmer N, Kaiser TE, et al. Combination therapy in liver transplant recipients with hepatitis B virus without hepatitis B immune globulin. Dig Dis Sci 2007;52(10):2497–500.

96. Teperman LW, Poordad F, Bzowej N, et al. Randomized trial of emtricitabine/tenofovir disoproxil fumarate after hepatitis B immunoglobulin withdrawal after liver transplantation. Liver Transpl 2013;19(6):594–601.

97. Grellier L, Mutimer D, Ahmed M, et al. Lamivudine prophylaxis against reinfection in liver transplantation for hepatitis B cirrhosis. Lancet 1996;348(9036):1212–5.

98. Malkan G, Cattral MS, Humar A, et al. Lamivudine for hepatitis B in liver transplantation: a single-center experience. Transplantation 2000;69(7):1403–7.

99. Mutimer D, Dusheiko G, Barrett C, et al. Lamivudine without HBIg for prevention of graft reinfection by hepatitis B: long-term follow-up. Transplantation 2000;70(5):809–15.

100. Yoshida H, Kato T, Levi DM, et al. Lamivudine monoprophylaxis for liver transplant recipients with non-replicating hepatitis B virus infection. Clin Transplant 2007;21(2):166–71.

101. Lo CM, Liu CL, Lau GK, et al. Liver transplantation for chronic hepatitis B with lamivudine-resistant YMDD mutant using add-on adefovir dipivoxil plus lamivudine. Liver Transpl 2005;11(7):807–13.

102. Fox AN, Terrault NA. The option of HBIG-free prophylaxis against recurrent HBV. J Hepatol 2012;56(5):1189–97.

103. Wadhawan MG, Gupta S, Vij V, et al. Living related liver transplant (LRLT) in HBV DNA negative cirrhosis without hepatitis B immune globulin (HBIG). Hepatol Int 2011;5:38. (Abstract).

104. Tan J, Lok AS. Antiviral therapy for pre- and post-liver transplantation patients with hepatitis B. Liver Transpl 2007;13(3):323–6.

105. Perrillo R, Hann HW, Mutimer D, et al. Adefovir dipivoxil added to ongoing lamivudine in chronic hepatitis B with YMDD mutant hepatitis B virus. Gastroenterology 2004;126(1):81–90.

Hepatitis Delta: The Rediscovery

Mario Rizzetto, MD[a],*, Seyed Moayed Alavian, MD[b]

KEYWORDS

- Hepatitis D (delta) • Hepatitis D (delta) virus • HDV epidemiology • HDV transmission
- HDV drug addicts • HDV rediscovery

KEY POINTS

- Control of hepatitis B Virus worldwide is diminishing the circulation of hepatitis D virus (HDV).
- The epidemic of HDV in southern Europe in the 1980s has been brought under control; however, HDV is returning to Europe through immigration from areas where this infection remains endemic.
- The prevalence of HDV remains high and has a major medical impact in the poorest countries of the world and in many areas of the developing world.
- Although forgotten in the Western world, hepatitis D has not disappeared but remains an important medical issue, in particular in drug addicts.

INTRODUCTION
The Virus and its Biology

The 1970s were a time of excitement in hepatology. The discovery of the hepatitis B virus (HBV) at the end of the 1960s provided the key to unravel the mysteries of viral hepatitis; by the middle of the 1970s, hepatitis A was discovered and diagnostics were developed for hepatitis A and B.

A few years later, by simple medical scrutiny, a novel hepatitis agent was unexpectedly discovered in association with HBV infection. In the mid-1970s, in Torino, Italy, clinical and immunologic discrepancies led to the recognition of a new antigen-antibody system named delta in carriers of the hepatitis B surface antigen (HBsAg). The new reactivity was initially thought to be an antigen of HBV but its true nature emerged at the end of the 1970s from studies in chimpanzees at the National Institute of Health in the United States.[1] From the different expression in the liver of animals naive to HBV and in animals carrying HBsAg, both inoculated with the same HBsAg-positive serum containing delta, it became clear that the delta antigen, rather than being a component of the HBV, was the hallmark of a new defective RNA virus

[a] Division of Gastroenterology, University of Torino, Molinette, c.so Bramante 88, Torino 10126, Italy; [b] Middle East Liver Diseases Center (MELD Center), PO Box 14155/3651, Teheran, Iran
* Corresponding author. Division Gastroenterology, Az. Osp. Città della Salute e della Scienza di Torino, c.so Bramante 88, Torino 10126, Italy.
E-mail address: mario.rizzetto@unito.it

Clin Liver Dis 17 (2013) 475–487
http://dx.doi.org/10.1016/j.cld.2013.05.007
1089-3261/13/$ – see front matter © 2013 Elsevier Inc. All rights reserved.

requiring HBV for its own infection.[2] The new virus received the name of hepatitis D virus (HDV). In the 30 years that followed its discovery, the unique virology of HDV and its interplay with HBV have been elucidated.[3] It is the smallest animal virus possessing a circular RNA genome made up of only 1700 bases; its circular structure is driven by intramolecular base pairing into a rodlike conformation; it contains a ribozyme (ie, an RNA segment that retains the genetic information but is also able to self-cleave the viral RNA[4]); the ribozyme is essential to HDV replication, which occurs by a rolling-circle mechanism similar to the viroids of plants.[5]

The limited genetic capacity of HDV is not sufficient to code for enzymatic functions of its own; thus the initial enigma was how HDV is replicated.

Transcriptional experiments using low-dose amanitin,[3] a toxin that blocks the transcription of RNA polymerase, have shown that HDV RNA is replicated by the host cell polymerases, raising the question of how mammalian RNA polymerases that only accept DNA could replicate an RNA molecule. To explain this puzzle, it is postulated that the host RNA polymerases are deceived by the rodlike conformation of native HDV (resembling double-stranded DNA) to copy the viral RNA as if it were endogenous DNA.[3] Thus HDV turns to its advantage the replicative machinery of the infected host and needs HBV only for the HBsAg coat necessary for virion assembly and for the binding to hepatocytes; the corollary is that there is no specific enzymatic function of the virus to target for therapy, such as the polymerases and proteases of HBV and hepatitis C virus (HCV), and its synthesis is not influenced by the level of HBV DNA in serum.

The Current Perception of the Epidemiology of HDV

Assays for the antibody to HDV (anti-HD) as the serologic signature of HDV infection were developed soon after the discovery of the virus and became available commercially in 1984, expediting epidemiologic surveys. At the end of the 1980s, data collected throughout the decade suggested that no less than 5% of HBsAg carriers worldwide were also infected with the HDV, corresponding with about 15,000,000 individuals, and that dual HBV-HDV infection was usually associated with a severe and rapidly progressive liver disease resistant to treatment.[6]

Since then, the global scenario of HBV has distinctly changed. Vaccination, public health measures against acquired immunodeficiency syndrome (AIDS), and improvements in hygienic conditions have increasingly and efficiently controlled the spread of HBV in developed countries; by depriving the HDV of the biological substrate necessary to its propagation, the containment of HBV has led to the simultaneous decline of hepatitis D in all areas of the industrialized world where the infection was endemic in the 1980s. The reduction was so profound in southern Europe that it led at the end of the 1990s to the hypothesis that HDV infection was on the way to eradication and that hepatitis D would soon be cancelled from the list of communicable disease.[7]

Optimism has been premature. First, hepatitis D is reviving in Europe, where immigrants are reintroducing the disease. Second, the apparent absence of HDV in many developing areas was largely caused by lack of information; new attention and availability of diagnostics are showing that hepatitis D remains a major health problem throughout the world. Third, although the decline of HDV in industrialized countries is genuine, the extent of its decline is concealed by diminished testing because of the perception that hepatitis D is no longer a significant medical problem.

The current debate is whether HDV is returning or hepatitis D is simply a forgotten disease on the way to rediscovery.[8] To understand the issue, this article discusses the epidemiologic changes in the developed world in the last 30 years, the problem and the degree of alertness in the developing countries, and the current standing in drug addicts, the population that bears the highest medical brunt of the infection in the Western world.

THE EPIDEMIOLOGIC SCENARIO IN EUROPE

Consistent epidemiologic studies were carried out in the 1980s in Western countries, primarily in southern Europe where the prevalence of HBV was high.[9,10] The epidemiology of HDV could not be assessed following the parameters of HBV infection; testing for HDV in acute HBsAg hepatitis as a measure of the incidence of HDV (ie, acute hepatitis D) was unreliable because, in the acute setting, expression of HDV markers is often weak and elusive and does not persist after the clearance of the HBsAg; likewise, prevalence studies for anti-HD in blood donors, who usually represent the reference population for serologic surveys of blood-borne infections, were unrewarding because HDV superinfection results in chronic hepatitis D and a sickness status that precludes blood donation.

Consistent data were obtained when the analysis was addressed by medical categories. In southern Europe, HDV was endemic and an important cause of chronic hepatitis leading to cirrhosis; in North America and northern Europe, the infection was largely confined to intravenous drug addicts, in whom it was a major cause of severe and fulminant HBsAg hepatitis.[11]

Risk factors were the carriage of HBsAg, parenteral exposure to blood, sexual promiscuity, and living in unhygienic and overcrowded household conditions.[9,10]

The Decline of HDV

At the end of the 1980s, the prevalence of HDV started to diminish in Europe. In Italy, anti-HD in HBsAg carriers with liver disease diminished from 24.6% in 1983 to 8% in 1997[12,13]; the circulation of HDV had already consistently diminished at the time of the introduction of universal vaccination against HBV in 1991, because of behavioral changes and sexual restrictions fostered by the fear of AIDS and because of diminished natality and consequent reduction of family size.

Declines of HDV occurred in the 1990s throughout the Mediterranean and in Taiwan. In Turkey, the overall rates of anti-HD in chronic hepatitis and cirrhosis decreased from 29% to 12% and from 38% and 27%, respectively,[14] and in Taiwan the incidence of HDV as a cause of superinfection diminished from 23.7% to 4.2% from 1983 to 1996.[15]

Infection with HDV also declined in areas of eastern Europe that enforced better public health measures and started HBV vaccination. A decrease from 47.6% to 15.4% in the prevalence of anti-HD in patients with HBsAg-positive cirrhosis was reported in Belarus from 1991 to 1997[16]; among institutionalized children with chronic hepatitis B in southeast Romania, the prevalence of HDV declined from 33% in the decade 1990 to 2000 to 21% in the decade 2000 to 2009[17]; in a recent population study in sub-Carpathian and southeast Romania, no HDV case was found in 2851 people examined.[18]

The Return of HDV

Since the end of the last century, HDV has not declined further in western Europe; although the major epidemic of HDV of the 1970s to 1980s was brought under control, the residual health burden of hepatitis D has remained stable in the last 10 years. In 1386 HBsAg carriers studied in Italy in 2006 to 2007, the overall prevalence of anti-HD has remained 8.1% with no further downtrend; among the incident cases the prevalence was 14.3%, suggesting a new wave of HDV-infected people.[19]

In London, United Kingdom, anti-HD has been detected in about 8.5% of HBsAg carriers between 2000 and 2006.[20] In Hannover, Germany, the prevalence of the infection declined from 18.6% to 6.8% in the period from 1992 to 1997, but anti-HD increased in the past decade, with 8% to 14% of the HBsAg carriers being positive from 1999 onward.[21] Both in the United Kingdom and in Germany, most HDV carriers are migrants from eastern Europe, Africa, the Middle East, and Turkey; in France, HDV infection is seen predominantly in people from northern Africa.[22] Contemporary data indicate that migration from areas where HDV remains endemic is reconstituting a reservoir of HDV infections in Europe (**Table 1**).

Clinical Changes

With the decline of HDV, the clinical scenario of hepatitis D has also changed. Although most patients with hepatitis D observed in Italy in the 1980s had a florid chronic hepatitis and cirrhosis was seen in fewer than 20% of cases, by the end of the 1990s the proportion of cirrhosis residual to burnt-out inflammation had increased to 70%.[23] In Barcelona, Spain, patients recruited from 1983 to 1995 were younger, had acquired HDV mainly by coinfection, and were often intravenous drug addicts and coinfected by HCV and HIV.[24] In contrast, patients recruited from 1996 to 2008 were older, with a higher proportion of immigrants, most presenting with chronic hepatitis D acquired by superinfection.

THE EPIDEMIOLOGIC SCENARIO OUTSIDE EUROPE
The Scenario in the 1980s to 1990s

The largest epidemiologic studies in the 1990s were promoted by major health institutions interested in extreme scenarios.

The US Centers for Disease Control and Prevention, the French Institute Pasteur, and the Kashmir Institute of Medical Science investigated outbreaks of fulminant hepatitis occurring in the Amazon basin,[25,26] the Central African Republic,[27] and the Himalayan foothills.[28] These epidemics resulted from the rapid spreading of HDV against a background of diffuse HBV infection in populations with poor hygienic conditions and overcrowding; those affected were mainly children and adolescents who had acquired HBV in infancy, and mortality was high.

Many small studies were carried out to establish local prevalences of HDV. However, there was no systematic or comprehensive survey; most studies were based on few patients with disparate clinical features. In many countries there was no facility or resource for local testing for HDV. It nevertheless became clear that the prevalence of HDV was not a simple replica of the HBV scenario, because the ratio of HDV to HBV varied widely throughout the world.

Most puzzling was the discrepancy between the high prevalence of endemic HDV in Taiwan and Okinawa and the very low prevalence in nearby Japan and Korea despite a

Table 1		
Prevalence of immigrants among individuals with HDV infection in Europe		
	% Immigrants, Origin	**Reference**
Greece	65, from the Balkans, central Asia, Africa	17
Hannover	80, from Turkey, eastern Europe	21
London	85, from eastern Europe, Asia, Africa	20
Spain	28, from Africa, eastern Europe, South America	24

The situation is similar and more emblematic in the United States. Although no further attention was apparently paid to HDV since the late 1980s, recent studies are urging reconsideration. In 2005, Bialek and colleagues[67] reported a 34.5% prevalence of HDV infection among 58 cases of acute HBsAg hepatitis reported in 2000; all the patients coinfected with HDV were drug addicts. In 2010, Kucirka and colleagues[68] compared the prevalence of anti-HD between 48 drug addicts in Baltimore with chronic HBsAg infection collected in 1988 to 1989 and 38 such patients collected in 2005 to 2006; the prevalence of anti-HD increased from 25% in the early cohort to 50% in the recent cohort.

In a retrospective review of 1296 chronic HBV carriers at California Pacific Medical Center,[17] 82 patients were positive for HDV (6.3%), and 34% were also infected with HCV. Sixty-three percent of the patients were born in North America, and most of the others came from south and east Asia and the Middle East; 23% of the patients reported a history of drug use.

Although these studies include a limited number of patients and were conducted too far away to draw nationwide conclusions, they nevertheless provide a warning that HDV is found from Baltimore to California not only in significant proportions of drug addicts but also in a more composite epidemiology including, as in Europe, immigrant populations.

SUMMARY

Hepatitis D is both returning and rediscovered. It is returning to western Europe through immigration. Immigrants account for the largest proportion of contemporary hepatitis D in the United Kingdom, Germany, and France; in Italy, Spain, and Greece they are reconstituting a reservoir of the infection, overtaking the decreasing and aging domestic patients with HDV. Their clinical presentation recapitulates the typical features of a florid hepatitis D seen in European patients in the 1970s to 1980s when HDV was endemic in southern Europe. Although the return of HDV is unlikely to have an impact in domestic European populations vaccinated against HBV, knowledge of the problem will be useful to enforce more vigilance and public health measures among newcomers.

Hepatitis D is being rediscovered in the developing world and in the United States. In the developing world, increased diagnostic facilities are raising awareness that HDV remains endemic in many countries; efforts are underway to map the infection at local levels and improve the medical alert to hepatitis D.

In the United States it is generally thought that HDV has gone and hepatitis D is no longer a problem; this perception seems to derive from lack of testing rather than from updated serologic surveys. Awareness of hepatitis D in the country has recently been revived, pointing to drug addicts as the major, but possibly not the only, residual reservoir of HDV in the country. Although long forgotten, HDV has not gone and should be considered in all patients with HBsAg liver disease, in particular in those with a history of drug addiction.[69]

REFERENCES

1. Rizzetto M. Hepatitis D: thirty years after. J Hepatol 2009;50:1043–50.
2. Rizzetto M. The delta agent. Hepatology 1983;3:729–37.
3. Taylor JM. Structure and replication of hepatitis delta virus RNA. Curr Top Microbiol Immunol 2006;307:1–23.
4. Been MD. HDV ribozymes. Curr Top Microbiol Immunol 2006;307:47–65.
5. Flores R, Ruiz-Ruiz S, Serra P. Viroids and hepatitis delta virus. Semin Liver Dis 2012;32:201–10.

6. Rizzetto M, Ponzetto A, Forzani I. Hepatitis delta virus as a global health problem. Vaccine 1990;(Suppl 8):S10–4 [discussion: S21–3].

7. Gaeta GB, Stroffolini T, Chiaramonte M, et al. Chronic hepatitis D: a vanishing disease? An Italian multicenter study. Hepatology 2000;32:824–7.

8. Rizzetto M. Delta hepatitis: forgotten, but not gone. Curr Hepat Rep 2010;9: 239–42.

9. Rizzetto M, Ponzetto A, Forzani I. Epidemiology of hepatitis delta virus: overview. Prog Clin Biol Res 1991;364:1–20.

10. Rizzetto M, Hadziyannis S, Hannson B, et al. Hepatitis delta virus infection in the world: epidemiologic patterns and clinical expression. Gastroenterol Int 1992;5: 18–32.

11. Smedile A, Rizzetto M, Gerin JL. Advances in hepatitis D virus biology and disease. In: Boyer JL, Ockner RK, editors. Progress in liver disease, vol. XII. Philadelphia: WB Saunders; 1994. p. 157–75.

12. Smedile A, Lavarini C, Farci P, et al. Epidemiologic patterns of infection with the hepatitis B virus-associated delta agent in Italy. Am J Epidemiol 1983;117: 223–9.

13. Sagnelli E, Stroffolini T, Ascione A, et al. Decrease in HDV endemicity in Italy. J Hepatol 1997;26:20–4.

14. Değertekin H, Yalçın K, Yakut M, et al. Seropositivity for delta hepatitis in patients with chronic hepatitis B and liver cirrhosis in Turkey: a meta-analysis. Liver Int 2008;28:494–8.

15. Huo TI, Wu JC, Lin RY, et al. Decreasing hepatitis D virus infection in Taiwan: an analysis of contributory factors. J Gastroenterol Hepatol 1997;12:747–51.

16. Ciancio A, Rizzetto M. Clinical patterns, epidemiology and disease burden of hepatitis D virus chronic liver disease. In: Margolis H, Alter M, Liang T, et al, editors. 10th International Symposium on Viral Hepatitis and Liver Disease. London: International Medical Press; 2002. p. 271–5.

17. Rizzetto M, Ciancio A. Epidemiology of hepatitis D. Semin Liver Dis 2012;32: 211–9.

18. Voiculescu M, Iliescu L, Ionescu C, et al. A cross-sectional epidemiological study of HBV, HCV, HDV and HEV prevalence in the SubCarpathian and south-eastern regions of Romania. J Gastrointestin Liver Dis 2010;19:43–8.

19. Stroffolini T, Almasio PL, Sagnelli E, et al. Evolving clinical landscape of chronic hepatitis B: a multicenter Italian study. J Med Virol 2009;81:1999–2006.

20. Cross TJ, Rizzi P, Horner M, et al. The increasing prevalence of hepatitis delta virus (HDV) infection in south London. J Med Virol 2008;80:277–82.

21. Heidrich B, Deterding K, Tillmann HL, et al. Virological and clinical characteristics of delta hepatitis in central Europe. J Viral Hepat 2009;16:883–94.

22. Le Gal F, Castelneau C, Gault E, et al. Hepatitis D virus infection. Not a vanishing disease in Europe! Hepatology 2007;45:1332–3.

23. Rosina F, Conoscitore P, Cuppone R, et al. Changing pattern of chronic hepatitis D in southern Europe. Gastroenterology 1999;117:161–6.

24. Buti M, Homs M, Rodriguez-Frias F, et al. Clinical outcome of acute and chronic hepatitis delta over time: a long-term follow-up study. J Viral Hepat 2011;18: 434–42.

25. Buitrago B, Hadler SC, Popper H, et al. Epidemiologic aspects of Santa Marta hepatitis over a 40-year period. Hepatology 1986;6:1292–6.

26. Hadler SC, de Monzon M, Ponzetto A. An epidemic of severe hepatitis due to delta virus infection in Yupca Indians in Venezuela. Ann Intern Med 1984;100: 339–44.

27. Lesbordes JL, Ravisse P, Georges AJ, et al. Studies on the role of HDV in an outbreak of fulminant hepatitis in Bangui (Central African Republic). Prog Clin Biol Res 1987;234:451–9.
28. Khuroo MS, Zargar SA, Mahajan R, et al. An epidemic of hepatitis D in the foothills of the Himalayas in south Kashmir. J Hepatol 1988;7:151–6.
29. Kim HS, Kim SJ, Park HW, et al. Prevalence and clinical significance of hepatitis D virus co-infection in patients with chronic hepatitis B in Korea. J Med Virol 2011;83:1172–7.
30. Greenfield C, Farci P, Osidiana V, et al. Hepatitis delta virus infection in Kenya. Its geographic and tribal distribution. Am J Epidemiol 1986;123:416–23.
31. Flodgren E, Bengtsson S, Knutsson M, et al. Recent high incidence of fulminant hepatitis in Samara, Russia: molecular analysis of prevailing hepatitis B and D virus strains. J Clin Microbiol 2000;38:3311–6.
32. Børresen ML, Olsen OR, Ladefoged K, et al. Hepatitis D outbreak among children in a hepatitis B hyper-endemic settlement in Greenland. J Viral Hepat 2010;17:162–70.
33. Davaalkham D, Ojima T, Uehara R, et al. Hepatitis deltavirus infection in Mongolia: analyses of geographic distribution, risk factors and disease severity. Am J Trop Med Hyg 2006;75:365–9.
34. Tsatsralt-Od B, Takahashi M, Endo K, et al. Infection with hepatitis A, B, C and delta viruses among patients with acute hepatitis in Mongolia. J Med Virol 2006;78:542–50.
35. Makuwa M, Mintsa-Ndong A, Souquière S, et al. Prevalence and molecular diversity of hepatitis B virus and hepatitis delta virus in urban and rural populations in northern Gabon in central Africa. J Clin Microbiol 2009;47:2265–8.
36. Foupouapouognigni Y, Noah DN, Sartre MT, et al. High prevalence and predominance of hepatitis delta virus genotype 1 infection in Cameroon. J Clin Microbiol 2011;49:1162–4.
37. Nwokediuko SC, Ijeoma U. Seroprevalence of antibody to HDV in Nigerians with hepatitis B virus-related liver diseases. Niger J Clin Pract 2009;12:439–42.
38. Mansour W, Malick FZ, Sidiya A, et al. Prevalence, risk factors, and molecular epidemiology of hepatitis B and hepatitis delta virus in pregnant women and in patients in Mauritania. J Med Virol 2012;84:1186–98.
39. Bayan K, Yilmaz S, Tuzun Y, et al. Epidemiological and clinical aspects of liver cirrhosis in adult patients living in southeastern Anatolia: leading role of HBV in 505 cases. Hepatogastroenterology 2007;54:2198–202.
40. Bahcecioglu IH, Aygun C, Gozel N, et al. Prevalence of hepatitis delta virus (HDV) infection in chronic hepatitis B patients in eastern Turkey: still a serious problem to consider. J Viral Hepat 2011;18:518–24.
41. Khan A, Kurbanov F, Tanaka Y, et al. Epidemiological and clinical evaluation of hepatitis B, hepatitis C, and delta hepatitis viruses in Tajikistan. J Med Virol 2008;80:268–76.
42. Amini N, Alavian SM, Kabir A, et al. Prevalence of hepatitis D in the eastern Mediterranean region: systematic review and meta analysis. Hepat Mon 2013;13:e8210.
43. Abbas Z, Jafri W, Raza S, et al. Scenario in the Asia-Pacific region. World J Gastroenterol 2010;16:554–62.
44. Hyams KC, al-Arabi MA, al-Tagani AA, et al. Epidemiology of hepatitis B in the Gezira region of Sudan. Am J Trop Med Hyg 1989;40:200–6.
45. Seetlani NK, Abbas Z, Raza S, et al. Prevalence of hepatitis D in HBsAg positive patients visiting liver clinics. J Pak Med Assoc 2009;59:434–7.

46. Darwish MA, Shaker M, Raslan O, et al. Hepatitis B & D viral infections among schistosomal patients in Egypt. J Egypt Public Health Assoc 1992;67:549–63.

47. Darwish MA, Shaker M, Raslan OS, et al. Delta virus infection in Egypt. J Egypt Public Health Assoc 1992;67:147–61.

48. Ramia S, el-Hazmi MA, Vivian PA, et al. Delta agent infection in Riyadh, Saudi Arabia. Trans R Soc Trop Med Hyg 1987;81:317–8.

49. Alavian SM, Alavian SH. Hepatitis D virus infection; Iran, Middle East and central Asia. Hepat Mon 2005;5:137–43.

50. Alizadeh AH, Ranjbar M, Tehrani AS, et al. Seroprevalence of hepatitis D virus and its risk factors in the west of Iran. J Microbiol Immunol Infect 2010;43:519–23.

51. Amini S, Mahmoodi MF, Andalibi S, et al. Seroepidemiology of hepatitis B, delta and HIV infections in Hamadan province of Iran. J Trop Med Hyg 1993;96: 277–87.

52. Hajiani E, Hashemi SJ, Jalali F. Seroprevalence of delta hepatitis in patients with chronic hepatitis B and its clinical impact in Khuzestan province, southwest Iran. Hepat Mon 2009;9:287–92.

53. Malekzadeh R, Borhanmanesh F. Prevalence of HDV in asymptomatic healthy carrier of HBV in Iran. Iran J Med Sci 1989;14:33–8.

54. Scott DA, Burans JP, al-Ouzeib HD, et al. A seroepidemiological survey of viral hepatitis in the Yemen Arab Republic. Trans R Soc Trop Med Hyg 1990;84: 288–91.

55. Ramia S, El-Zaatari M, Sharara AI, et al. Current prevalence of hepatitis delta virus (HDV) infection and the range of HDV genotypes in Lebanon. Epidemiol Infect 2007;135:959–62.

56. Abbatte EA, Fox E, Said S, et al. Ethnic differences in the prevalence of hepatitis delta agent in Djibouti. Trans R Soc Trop Med Hyg 1989;83:107–8.

57. Toukan AU, Abu-el-Rub OA, Abu-Laban SA, et al. The epidemiology and clinical outcome of hepatitis D virus (delta) infection in Jordan. Hepatology 1987;7:1340–5.

58. Aceti A, Paparo BS, Celestino D, et al. Sero-epidemiology of hepatitis delta virus infection in Somalia. Trans R Soc Trop Med Hyg 1989;83:399–400.

59. Aceti A, Mohamed OM, Paparo BS, et al. High prevalence of anti-hepatitis delta virus antibody in chronic liver disease in Somalia. Trans R Soc Trop Med Hyg 1991;85:541–2.

60. Jacobson IM, Dienstag JL, Werner BG, et al. Epidemiology and clinical impact of hepatitis D virus (delta) infection. Hepatology 1985;5:188–91.

61. Ponzetto A, Seeff LB, Buskell-Bales Z, et al. Hepatitis B markers in United States drug addicts with special emphasis on the delta hepatitis virus. Hepatology 1984;4:1111–5.

62. Lettau LA, McCarthy JG, Smith MH, et al. Outbreak of severe hepatitis due to delta and hepatitis B viruses in parenteral drug abusers and their contacts. N Engl J Med 1987;317:1256–62.

63. Novick DM, Farci P, Croxson TS, et al. Hepatitis D virus and human immunode-ficiency virus antibodies in parenteral drug abusers who are hepatitis B surface antigen positive. J Infect Dis 1988;158:795–803.

64. Genné D, Rossi I. Hepatitis delta in Switzerland: a silent epidemic. Swiss Med Wkly 2011;141:w13176.

65. Soriano V, Grint D, d'Arminio Monforte A, et al. Hepatitis delta in HIV-infected individuals in Europe. AIDS 2011;25:1987–92.

66. Ionescu B, Mihăescu G, Hepatitis B. C and D coinfection in HIV-infected pa-tients: prevalence and progress. Roum Arch Microbiol Immunol 2011;70: 129–33.

67. Bialek SR, Bower WA, Mottram K, et al. Risk factors for hepatitis B in an outbreak of hepatitis B and D among injection drug users. J Urban Health 2005;82: 468–78.
68. Kucirka LM, Farzadegan H, Feld JJ, et al. Prevalence, correlates, and viral dynamics of hepatitis delta among injection drug users. J Infect Dis 2010;202: 845–52.
69. Holmberg SD, Ward JW. Hepatitis delta: seek and ye shall find. J Infect Dis 2010;202:822–4.

Hepatitis B in HIV-Infected Patients

Vincent Soriano, MD, PhD*, Eva Poveda, PhD, Eugenia Vispo, MD,
Pablo Barreiro, MD, PhD

KEYWORDS

- HBV-HIV coinfection • HBV vaccine • Tenofovir • Lamivudine
- Hepatocellular carcinoma • Liver fibrosis • Drug resistance

KEY POINTS

- Assessment of HBV status is warranted in all HIV patients.
- HBV vaccination should be given to all susceptible HIV patients.
- Treatment of HIV including anti-HBV active agents should be given to all HIV-HBV coinfected individuals, regardless of CD4 counts.
- Although tenofovir is the drug of choice in HIV-HBV coinfected individuals, lamivudine as the only active anti-HBV agent may be considered in certain scenarios.
- Periodic assessment of liver fibrosis using noninvasive tools is warranted in all HIV-HBV coinfected patients.
- Periodic screening for hepatocellular carcinoma should be performed in cirrhotics.

EPIDEMIOLOGY

Of the nearly two billion people have been infected with the hepatitis B virus (HBV), nearly 15% remain chronically positive for the HBV surface antigen (HBsAg). Overall, progressive liver disease, including development of liver cancer, occurs lifelong in 15% to 40% of chronic HBsAg carriers in the absence of antiviral treatment.[1] As in the case of HIV, HBV is mainly transmitted by perinatal, parenteral, and sexual contacts, which explains why HIV and HBV coinfection is relatively common.[2] Current estimates place the prevalence of chronic hepatitis B (CHB) among HIV-infected patients between 5% and 20%. Thus, 2 to 4 million out of 35 million people living with HIV worldwide have CHB.[2,3] In some regions in sub-Saharan Africa and Southeast Asia, HBsAg can be found in up to 15% to 20% of the HIV population.[4] In Europe, nearly 10% of HIV-infected individuals have CHB, more than 100-fold the rate in the general

Department of Infectious Diseases, Hospital Carlos III, calle Sinesio delgado 10, Madrid 28029, Spain
* Corresponding author.
E-mail address: vsoriano@dragonet.es

Clin Liver Dis 17 (2013) 489–501
http://dx.doi.org/10.1016/j.cld.2013.05.008
1089-3261/13/$ – see front matter © 2013 Elsevier Inc. All rights reserved.

population.[2] In the United States, it is estimated that half of HIV-positive (+) persons have been exposed to HBV and, therefore, exhibit markers of spontaneously self-limited HBV infection (HBV core antibodies [HbcAb] with or without HBV surface antibodies [HbsAb]) or have current HBsAg+ infection.[5]

Across several studies, the prevalence of HBsAg+ after HIV diagnosis has remained relatively unchanged since the year 2000, which means that recommendations for HBV vaccination to high-risk populations need to be refreshed and implemented. In developing countries, HBV is mainly transmitted in the perinatal period from HBsAg+ mothers, in early childhood from infected peers, or in early youth by heterosexual contact.[4] In Western countries, HBV vaccination campaigns have halted HBV infection of newborns and infants, so that most cases occur among youngsters, particularly in men who have sex with men (MSM).[6]

The distribution of 10 HBV genotypes, named with letters from A to J, differs in distinct geographic regions (**Box 1**).[1] HBV genotype A predominates in Northern Europe and North America, genotypes B and C are common in Asia and genotype D is mostly found in the Mediterranean basin and Eastern Europe. This distribution may in part be because HBV genotype A is more frequently acquired through sexual contact, whereas HBV genotype D is more frequently found in injecting drug users (IDUs).[7] The genotype of HBV may determine the course of CHB because HBV genotypes C and D are associated with faster progression to cirrhosis and liver cancer, whereas HBV genotypes A and B may be more susceptible to interferon (IFN) therapy.[8] In the case of HIV+ patients with CHB living in Europe, HBV genotype A is the most prevalent; it is found in approximately three-quarters of HIV-HBV coinfected individuals. In Southern Europe, HBV genotype D is equally prevalent to genotype A in this population.[7]

CLINICAL OUTCOME

Most individuals exposed to HBV ($\approx 85\%$) attain HBsAg seroconversion within the first 6 months, and develop HBcAb+ with or without HBsAb+. These patients have resolved, but not cured, HBV infection because integrated, episomal HBV-DNA remains in the hepatocytes. If the patient experiences potent immune suppression for any reason, HBV reactivation may occur.[9]

Box 1 Peculiarities of HBV according to genotype	
Genotype	**Main Characteristics**
A	Often HBV early antigen (HBeAg)+ and high viral load; good susceptibility to IFN
B	Good susceptibility to IFN
C	More often HBeAg-positive; increased risk of hepatocellular carcinoma
D	Often HBeAg-negative; poor susceptibility to IFN; more frequent delta superinfection
E	Widely prevalent in Africa
F	Prevalent in Central and South America
G	In 10% to 20% of HIV+ patients in North America and Western Europe; poor susceptibility to IFN; frequent coinfection with other genotypes; faster liver fibrosis progression
H	Prevalent in Central and South America
I	Initially reported in Laos and Vietnam; more recently in India; complex A/G/C recombinant nature
J	Recently reported in Japan; closer to orangutan HBV

Patients with HBsAg detectable in serum for longer than 6 months are considered to have CHB. During the first years of CHB, HBeAg is generally positive, which is associated with elevated serum HBV-DNA levels (>20,000 IU/mL). HBeAg seroconversion occurs at a rate of 8% to 12% per year, followed by normalization in liver enzymes, aspartate transaminase (AST) and alanine transaminase (ALT), and decline or even suppression in HBV-DNA levels (inactive HBsAg carrier state).[10] This event occurs more frequently with older age, high ALT, and in HBV genotype B. However, in 10% to 30% of HBeAg-negative patients, ALT is elevated and serum HBV-DNA levels are greater than 2000 IU/mL. These individuals usually harbor and replicate HBV core or precore mutants.[11,12] Spontaneous HBsAg clearance is a rare event and occurs at a rate of 0.5% per year in CHB. It is generally preceded by low or undetectable (resolved) HBV.[10]

The natural history of CHB is often more complex than described above. Patients can exhibit a wide range of hepatic damage with diverse degrees of inflammation and fibrosis.[13] Final events are cirrhosis, end-stage liver disease (ESLD), and hepatocellular carcinoma (HCC). Factors associated with fatal outcomes in CHB are male gender, black or Asian race, family history of liver cancer, high HBV-DNA levels, and HBeAg+.[14,15] Compared with HBV-monoinfected individuals, HIV-HBV coinfected patients have lower chances for spontaneous HBeAg and HBsAg clearance. Serum HBV-DNA levels are more elevated, which may in part explain the faster progression to ESLD and HCC characteristically seen in coinfected patients.[16-20]

Following the advent and broader use of highly active antiretroviral therapy (HAART), opportunistic complications have declined dramatically. However, liver-related complications are on the rise in patients coinfected with hepatitis viruses, mainly B and C.[21-23] Current knowledge suggests that treatment of both HIV and HBV may prevent or slow down the development of hepatic complications in coinfected patients.[22,24] Accordingly, most HIV treatment guidelines recommend earlier HIV and HBV therapy in HIV-HBV coinfection regardless of CD4 counts.[25-27] This goal can be easily accomplished using oral drugs with dual antiviral activity (ie, lamivudine [LAM], emtricitabine [FTC], or tenofovir [TDF]).[28] The enhanced risk of liver toxicity of antiviral agents, particularly among cirrhotic HIV-HBV coinfected patients,[29-31] should not preclude prescription of HIV plus HBV therapy, although antivirals with the safest liver profile should be preferred.[32] The patient should be warned against stopping HAART with anti-HBV drugs for any reason because abrupt resumption of HBV replication may lead to a flare in liver enzymes and even fulminant hepatic failure.[32]

DIAGNOSIS

All HIV-infected persons must be tested for HBV markers of current (HBsAg+) or past infection (HBcAb+ with or without HBsAb+). Testing must be refreshed in patients with special features such as unexplained ALT elevations, visits or living in endemic areas, household contact with HBsAg+ persons, IDUs, multiple sexual contacts, history of sexually transmitted diseases, MSM, prison inmates, pregnant women, and chronic HCV individuals.[33]

Because fulminant viral hepatitis is more common in patients with underlying chronic liver disease, hepatitis A virus (HAV) vaccination is recommended for all patients with CHB and negative HAV-Ab.[34] Given the overlapping transmission routes, all HIV-HBV coinfected patients should be tested for the presence of concomitant hepatitis C virus (HCV) and/or hepatitis D (or delta) virus (HDV) infection.[27,34]

ALT values, HBV genotype, HBeAg, and serum HBV-DNA levels need to be assessed at baseline in all patients with CHB so that therapeutic decisions can be made and the best treatment option selected. If any antiviral, liver enzymes are started in treatment, the HBeAg, HBsAg, and HBV-DNA levels should be monitored every 3 to 12 months. The extent of liver fibrosis should be checked at baseline and, ideally, every 6 months using noninvasive tests such as transient elastometry, which is currently the most reliable and feasible tool to discriminate between advanced and minimal or absent liver fibrosis, especially in HIV-HBV coinfected individuals.[35] In patients with advanced liver fibrosis, periodic screening for liver cancer, including serum alpha-fetoprotein, and ultrasonography every 6 months is warranted. Some evidence suggests that HIV individuals are at greater risk for HCC even in the absence of cirrhosis. This consideration particularly applies to African patients older than 20 years old, Asians older than 40 years old, persons with family history of HCC, and in the presence of high HBV-DNA levels (>2 million IU/mL). Screening for esophageal varices should be performed periodically in cirrhotics, and prophylaxis should be given with propranolol or other procedures accordingly.[34]

TREATMENT

In HIV patients with CHB, HBV therapy is indicated in all individuals with cirrhosis, CD4 counts less than 500 cells/μL, serum HBV-DNA greater than 2000 IU/mL, and/or elevated liver enzymes (**Fig. 1**).[31] Most experts recommend therapy irrespective of CD4 counts, given the accelerated progression of liver disease in HIV patients. For most patients, the best option is triple combination of antiretrovirals, including two reverse transcriptase inhibitors with anti-HBV activity; that is, TDF plus LAM or FTC. The coformulation of TDF-FTC (Truvada) makes this option the preferred one.

In very specific situations, peginterferon (pegIFN) alpha could be considered as therapy for CHB in coinfected patients. This is the case for patients unwilling to start HAART who have normal CD4 counts, HBeAg+, low HBV-DNA, elevated ALT, and lack of decompensated cirrhosis (**Fig. 2**).

Other treatment options, such as adefovir (ADV) or telbivudine (LdT) therapy, do not fit in the HIV setting due to the lack of or residual activity of these molecules against HIV and their relatively weak activity against HBV. Treatment with entecavir (ETV) may be needed in case TDF cannot be used, mostly due to kidney toxicity. Because

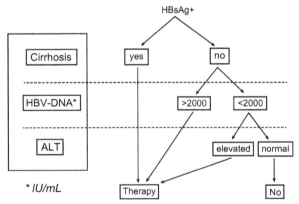

Fig. 1. Treatment indication for HBV infection in HIV-infected individuals. In patients with significant liver fibrosis (F2–F3), anti-HBV treatment might be considered even when serum HBV-DNA is greater than 2000 IU/mL and liver enzymes are not elevated. (*Adapted from* European AIDS Clinical Society Guidelines. Version 6.0. October 2011. Available at: http://www.europeanaidsclinicalsociety.org.)

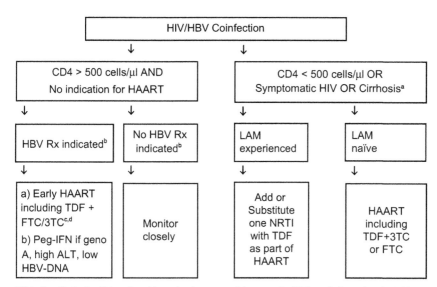

Fig. 2. Treatment of CHB infection in HIV+ individuals. NRTI, nucleos(t)ide reverse transcriptase inhibitors. (*Adapted from* European AIDS Clinical Society Guidelines. Version 6.0. October 2011. Available at: http://www.europeanaidsclinicalsociety.org.)

ETV displays weak activity against HIV and may select for resistance mutations, it should be administered only in the context of a fully suppressive HIV treatment.[36]

Oral anti-HBV drugs may select changes at the HBV polymerase, leading to loss of susceptibility to the corresponding drug and cross-resistance to other antivirals. Compared with HIV or HCV, HBV selects drug-resistant viral mutants more slowly, which largely depends on the longer half-life of infected hepatocytes carrying viral covalently closed circular DNA (cccDNA) virions.[37] Among the drugs used as HBV therapy, LAM has the lowest barrier for resistance, with emergence of drug-resistant mutants in 25% to 65% of patients treated for 1 to 5 years, respectively.[28,34] LdT selects drug-resistant mutant viruses at a rate of 20% within 2 years. This rate is approximately 29% for ADV at 5 years. The greatest barrier to resistance is exhibited by TDF and ETV. However, because ETV resistance is very rare in naïve individuals (<2% at 5 years), it may develop in nearly half of patients with previous LAM failure after 5 years of treatment.[38]

Changes in M204 I or V are usually responsible for LAM, FTC, and LdT resistance, whereas more changes (L180M plus M204V plus T250) are usually needed for ETV resistance. Accordingly, cross-resistance is almost universal with LAM, FTC, LdT, and to a lesser extent with ETV. There is some cross-resistance to ADV in the presence of A181S plus M204 I mutations in patients who have failed LAM therapy.[39,40] No mutations have been uniformly associated with significant loss of susceptibility to TDF in vivo, although anecdotal reports have pointed out that A194T in the context of LAM resistance mutations might account for TDF resistance in HBV (**Fig. 3**).[41]

Resistance to LAM in HBV is more common and develops faster in HIV-HBV coinfected patients, in part due to generally greater serum HBV-DNA levels.[42–44] Selection of LAM resistance in CHB is associated with poor outcomes, including the occurrence of liver enzyme flares, which occasionally may be life-threatening,[45,46] and precluding the success of rescue antiviral interventions due to cross-resistance with other antivirals. Additionally, because of overlapping polymerase and envelope genes in the HBV genome, LAM resistance mutations may result in changes in the HBsAg, causing diminished HBs antigen-antibody binding. This may translate into failure in diagnostic tests, vaccine escape, or both.[47–49] Finally, and to a lesser extent than in HIV, transmission of drug-resistant HBV strains has already been reported.[50–52] This latest finding seems currently restricted to LAM and has not been reported for other anti-HBV agents. Transmission of LAM-resistant HBV strains has been reported in up to 5% to 8% of newly diagnosed HBV patients.[53,54] This observation constitutes a further argument against the use of LAM as the only active drug against HBV in HIV-HBV coinfected patients.[43,44]

The current economic scenario, which affects both developing and developed countries, encourages exploration of the cheapest options for HBV therapy. Rethinking

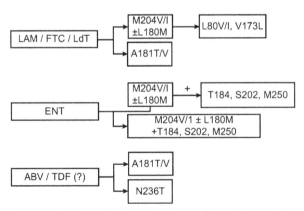

Fig. 3. Pathways of HBV resistance to oral drugs. ABV, abacavir; ENT, entecavir. (*Data from* Tenney D. Genotypic determinants and phenotypic properties of antiviral-resistant HBV variants: insight from entecavir resistance studies. Antivir Ther 2010;15:529–35.)

therapeutic strategies for HBV in response to economic constraints is always challenging because patient safety must be preserved.[55] The cost of LAM (1 to 2 US dollars per day), now available as generic drug, is much cheaper than the cost of TDF (10 to 12 US dollars per day) or ETV (15 US dollars per day). Moreover, although LAM is usually very well tolerated,[56] TDF may be associated with kidney tubular abnormalities,[57,58] which infrequently may lead to Fanconi syndrome[59] or, even more rarely, to overt renal insufficiency.[60] In HIV patients, prolonged TDF therapy has, in some cases, led to bone demineralization and increased risk of osteopenia and bone fractures.[61]

Besides the unaffordable cost of medications, another important limitation for the judicious use of antiviral medications in resource-limited settings is the high cost of HBV-DNA testing and of tools for liver fibrosis assessment, including liver biopsy. In this scenario, HBeAg negativity may be a good surrogate marker for low HBV-DNA levels and LAM as the only anti-HBV drug may be a good first-line option (**Fig. 4**A).[55,62,63] If HBV-DNA testing is available, LAM might be initially prescribed as long as HBV-DNA suppression is potent enough to prevent the selection of drug-resistant mutants. Patients with HBV-DNA levels less than 2000 IU/mL at week 24 of LAM therapy may be expected to attain complete viral suppression under this simple regimen within the following months.

In patients with high HBV-DNA ($>10^6$ IU/mL), or with positive HBeAg, a more potent regimen containing TDF should be initially used.[55,64] However, later on, when undetectable HBV-DNA is achieved, simplification to a cheaper regimen with LAM may be enough to sustain viral suppression (see **Fig. 4**B). Nevertheless, LAM would probably never be a good option in cirrhotic patients because an eventual virological failure may provoke liver decompensation.[64] Primary LAM resistance in individuals that acquired an HBV mutant at first infection seems to be rare.[50–52,65] Unless this phenomenon gains frequency in certain areas, LAM use in the scenarios described above should be discouraged.[53,54]

VACCINATION

Universal infant HBV vaccination was recommended by the World Health Organization in 1992.[66] HIV-infected adults without protective HBsAb titers should be vaccinated.

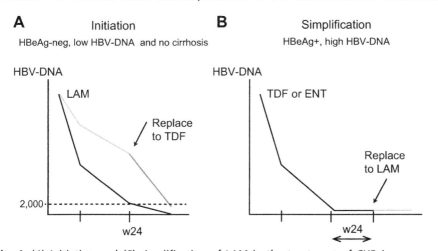

Fig. 4. (*A*) Initiation and (*B*) simplification of LAM in the treatment of CHB in resource-limited scenarios. (*Adapted from* Soriano V, McMahon B. Rethinking therapeutic strategies for hepatitis B. J Antimicrob Chemother, in press; with permission.)

The response rate and durability of the vaccine is poorer in HIV+ persons compared with HIV-negative persons,[67,68] and they are influenced by both CD4 counts and plasma HIV-RNA levels.[69] Accordingly, in patients with low CD4 counts (<200 cells/μL) and uncontrolled HIV replication, the success of HBV immunization is low. In these individuals, previous antiretroviral therapy for at least 6 months may increase HBV vaccine response rates.

Although most HIV guidelines still recommend an initial conventional HBV vaccination schedule, in the case of lack of achievement of protective anti-HBs titers (>10 mIU/mL) revaccination using double-dose and/or three to four injections (months 0, 1, 6, and 12) is frequently recommended.[70] Some protection from HBV vaccine may be expected even in the case of anti-HBs titers dropping to less than 10 mIU/mL.[71]

HDV

HDV infection only occurs in subjects with CHB because this agent requires HBsAg to complete replication at the hepatocyte. Approximately 5% of patients with CHB worldwide exhibit HDV coinfection, with large geographic disparities, peaking to 8% or higher in some areas of the Mediterranean basin, Eastern Europe, and Latin America.[72] The prevalence of HDV among HIV-HBV coinfected patients is approximately 15% in Western Europe.[73] It is going down because IDU has declined dramatically and HBV vaccination is broadly ensured in the HIV population.[74]

HDV coinfection causes CHB to run faster to ESLD and HCC.[75,76] The only approved treatment of HDV infection is pegIFN alpha, although less than 20% of patients attain sustained HDV-RNA suppression.[77,78] Improvement in liver histology has been noticed in patients who achieved sustained viral response after HDV therapy with IFN.[79] The addition of ribavirin, LAM, or ADV to pegIFN did not demonstrate any benefit in terms of response rate to pegIFN alone.[80–82] Ongoing studies are exploring the potential benefit of adding the newer, more potent, oral drugs TDF or ETV. Information on TDF is particularly appealing because earlier reports have already suggested some efficacy of the drug in HIV patients with HDV, particularly in those infected with HBV genotype A.[18,83] Duration of pegIFN therapy is flexible but should not be given for less than a year, considering extension based on initial biochemical and/or virological response and tolerance. In patients experiencing a significant HDV-RNA drop after 6 to 12 months of treatment, pegIFN should be maintained until complete HDV-RNA suppression is achieved. Because relapses are common, when possible, treatment should be extended until HBsAg loss is attained.[84] This circumstance, however, is rarely achieved. In patients with HDV and ESLD or HCC, liver transplantation should be strongly considered, especially in the absence of active HCV coinfection because liver transplant may cure HBV and HDV infection.[85]

REFERENCES

1. Te H, Jensen D. Epidemiology of hepatitis B and C viruses: a global overview. Clin Liver Dis 2010;14:1–21.
2. Konopnicki D, Mocroft A, de Wit S, et al. Hepatitis B and HIV: prevalence, AIDS progression, response to HAART and increased mortality in the EuroSIDA cohort. AIDS 2005;19:2117–25.
3. Kellerman S, Hanson D, McNaghten A, et al. Prevalence of chronic hepatitis B and incidence of acute hepatitis B infection in HIV-infected participants. J Infect Dis 2003;188:571–7.
4. Modi A, Feld J. Viral hepatitis and HIV in Africa. AIDS Rev 2007;9:25–39.

5. Chun H, Fieberg A, Hullsied K, et al. Epidemiology of hepatitis B virus infection in a US cohort of HIV-infected individuals during the past 20 years. Clin Infect Dis 2010;50:426–36.
6. Lavanchy D. Hepatitis B virus epidemiology, disease burden, treatment, and current and emerging prevention and control measures. J Viral Hepat 2004; 11:97–107.
7. Soriano V, Mocroft A, Peters L, et al. Predictors of hepatitis B virus genotype and viraemia in HIV-infected patients with chronic hepatitis B in Europe. J Antimicrob Chemother 2010;65:548–55.
8. Wong V, Sung J. Diagnosis and personalized management of hepatitis B including significance of genotypes. Curr Opin Infect Dis 2012;25:570–7.
9. Yeo W, Johnson P. Diagnosis, prevention and management of hepatitis B virus reactivation during anticancer therapy. Hepatology 2006;43:209–20.
10. McMahon B, Holck P, Bulkow L, et al. Serologic and clinical outcomes of 1536 Alaska natives chronically infected with hepatitis B virus. Ann Intern Med 2001; 135:759–68.
11. Chan H, Leung N, Hussain M, et al. Hepatitis B e antigen-negative chronic hepatitis B in Hong Kong. Hepatology 2000;31:763–8.
12. Grandjacques C, Pradat P, Stuyver L, et al. Rapid detection of genotypes and mutations in the pre-core promoter and the pre-core region of hepatitis B virus genome: correlation with viral persistence and disease severity. J Hepatol 2000; 33:430–9.
13. McMahon B. The natural history of chronic hepatitis B virus infection. Hepatology 2009;49(Suppl):45–55.
14. Iloeje U, Yang H, Su J, et al. Predicting cirrhosis risk based on the level of circulating hepatitis B virus viral load. Gastroenterology 2006;130:678–86.
15. Chen C, Yang H, Su J, et al. Risk of hepatocellular carcinoma across biological gradient of serum hepatitis B virus DNA level. JAMA 2006;295:65–73.
16. Puoti C, Torti C, Bruno R, et al. Natural history of chronic hepatitis B in co-infected patients. J Hepatol 2006;44:S65–70.
17. Walter S, Thein H, Amin J, et al. Trends in mortality after diagnosis of hepatitis B or C infection: 1992–2006. J Hepatol 2011;54:879–86.
18. Martín-Carbonero L, Teixeira T, Poveda E, et al. Clinical and virological outcomes in HIV-infected patients with chronic hepatitis B on long-term nucleos(t)ide analogues. AIDS 2011;25:73–9.
19. Clifford G, Rickenbach M, Polesel J, et al. Influence of HIV-related immunodeficiency on the risk of hepatocellular carcinoma. AIDS 2008;22:2135–41.
20. Thio C. Hepatitis B and human immunodeficiency virus coinfection. Hepatology 2009;49(Suppl):138–45.
21. Weber R, Sabin C, Friis-Moller N, et al. Liver-related deaths in persons with the human immunodeficiency virus: the D:A:D study. Arch Intern Med 2006;166: 1632–41.
22. Nikolopoulos G, Paraskevis D, Hatzitheodorou E, et al. Impact of hepatitis B virus infection on the progression of AIDS and mortality in HIV-infected individuals: a cohort study and meta-analysis. Clin Infect Dis 2009;48:1763–71.
23. Thio C, Seaberg E, Skolasky R, et al. HIV-1, hepatitis B virus, and risk of liver-related mortality in the Multicenter Cohort Study (MACS). Lancet 2002;360:1921–6.
24. Hoffmann C, Seaberg E, Young S, et al. Hepatitis B and long-term HIV outcomes in coinfected HAART recipients. AIDS 2009;23:1881–9.
25. DHHS. Panel on treatment of HIV-infected pregnant women and prevention of perinatal transmission. Recommendations for use of antiretroviral drugs in

pregnant HIV-1-infected women for maternal health and interventions to reduce perinatal HIV transmission in the United States. Available at: http://aidsinfo.nih. gov/contentfiles/lvguidelines/perinatalgl.pdf.

26. Thompson M, Aberg J, Hoy J, et al. Antiretroviral treatment of adult HIV infection: 2012 recommendations of the International Antiviral Society-USA panel. JAMA 2012;308:387–402.

27. European AIDS Clinical Society Guidelines. Version 6.0. October 2011. Available at: http://www.europeanaidsclinicalsociety.org.

28. Soriano V, Tuma P, Vispo E, et al. Hepatitis B in HIV patients: what is the current treatment and what are the challenges? J HIV Ther 2009;14(1):13–8.

29. Sulkowski M, Thomas D, Chaisson R, et al. Hepatotoxicity associated with antiretroviral therapy in adults infected with HIV and the role of hepatitis C or B virus infection. JAMA 2000;283:74–80.

30. Aceti A, Pasquazzi C, Zechini B, et al. Hepatotoxicity development during antiretroviral therapy containing protease inhibitors in patients with HIV: the role of hepatitis B and C virus infection. J Acquir Immune Defic Syndr 2002;29:41–8.

31. Soriano V, Puoti M, Garcia-Gascó P, et al. Antiretroviral drugs and liver injury. AIDS 2008;22:1–13.

32. Soriano V, Puoti M, Peters M, et al. Care of HIV patients with chronic hepatitis B: updated recommendations from the HIV-Hepatitis B virus international panel. AIDS 2008;22:1399–410.

33. Lok A, McMahon B. Chronic hepatitis B: update 2009. Hepatology 2009;50: 661–96.

34. European Association for the Study of the Liver. EASL Clinical Practice Guidelines: management of chronic hepatitis B. J Hepatol 2009;50:227–42.

35. Soriano V, Sheldon J, Ramos B, et al. Confronting chronic hepatitis B virus infection in HIV: new diagnostic tools and more weapons. AIDS 2006;20:451–3.

36. McMahon M, Jilek B, Brennan T, et al. The HBV drug entecavir - effects on HIV-1 replication and resistance. N Engl J Med 2007;356:2614–21.

37. Soriano V, Perelson A, Zoulim F. Why are there different dynamics in the selection of drug resistance in HIV and hepatitis B and C viruses? J Antimicrob Chemother 2008;62:1–4.

38. Known H, Lock M. Hepatitis B therapy. Gastroenterol Hepatol 2011;8:275–84.

39. Karatayli E, Karayalcin S, Karaaslan H, et al. A novel mutation pattern emerging during lamivudine treatment shows cross-resistance to adefovir dipivoxil treatment. Antivir Ther 2007;12:761–8.

40. Tenney D. Genotypic determinants and phenotypic properties of antiviral-resistant HBV variants: insight from entecavir resistance studies. Antivir Ther 2010;15:529–35.

41. Sheldon J, Camino N, Rodes B, et al. Selection of hepatitis B virus polymerase mutations in HIV coinfected patients treated with tenofovir. Antivir Ther 2005;10: 727–34.

42. Benhamou Y, Bochet M, Thibault V, et al. Long-term incidence of hepatitis B virus resistance to lamivudine in HIV-infected patients. Hepatology 1999;30: 1302–6.

43. Hoffmann C, Charalambous S, Martin D, et al. Hepatitis B virus infection and response to antiretroviral therapy (ART) in a South African ART program. Clin Infect Dis 2008;47:1479–85.

44. Soriano V, Rivas P, Nuñez M. Risks and benefits of using antiretroviral therapy in HIV-infected patients with chronic hepatitis B in developing regions. Clin Infect Dis 2008;47:1486–9.

45. Matthews G, Bartholomeusz A, Locarnini S. Characteristics of drug resistant HBV in an international collaborative study of HIV-HBV-infected individuals on extended lamivudine therapy. AIDS 2006;20:863–70.
46. Gouskos T, Wightman F, Chang J, et al. Severe hepatitis and prolonged hepatitis B virus-specific CD8 T-cell response after selection of hepatitis B virus YMDD variant in an HIV/hepatitis B virus co-infected patient. AIDS 2004;18: 1734–7.
47. Hsu C, Yeh C, Chang M, et al. Identification of a hepatitis B virus S gene mutant in lamivudine-treated patients experiencing HBsAg seroclearance. Gastroenterology 2007;132:543–50.
48. Sheldon J, Soriano V. Hepatitis B virus escape mutants induced by antiviral therapy. J Antimicrob Chemother 2008;61:766–8.
49. Martín-Carbonero L, Soriano V. New paradigms for treating hepatitis B in HIV/HBV co-infected patients. J Antimicrob Chemother 2010;65:379–82.
50. Thibault V, Aubron-Olivier C, Agut H, et al. Primary infection with a lamivudine-resistant hepatitis B virus. AIDS 2002;16:131–3.
51. Tuma P, Pineda J, Labarga P, et al. HBV primary drug resistance in newly diagnosed HIV-HBV-coinfected individuals in Spain. Antivir Ther 2011;16: 585–9.
52. Fujisaki S, Yokomaku Y, Shiino T, et al. Outbreak of infections by hepatitis B virus genotype A and transmission of genetic drug resistance in patients coinfected with HIV-1 in Japan. J Clin Microbiol 2011;49:1017–24.
53. Xu Z, Liu Y, Xu T, et al. Acute hepatitis B infection associated with drug resistant hepatitis B virus. J Clin Virol 2010;48:270–4.
54. Fung S, Mazulli T, El-Kashab M, et al. Lamivudine-resistant mutation among treatment-naïve hepatitis B patients is common and may be associated with treatment failure. American Association for the Study of Liver Diseases. 31 Oct-4 Nov 2008; San Francisco, CA, USA [Abstract 888].
55. Soriano V, McMahon B. Rethinking therapeutic strategies for hepatitis B. J Antimicrob Chemother, in press.
56. Lok A, Lai C, Leung N, et al. Long-term safety of lamivudine treatment in patients with chronic hepatitis B. Gastroenterology 2003;125:1714–22.
57. Labarga P, Barreiro P, Martin-Carbonero L, et al. Kidney tubular abnormalities in the absence of impaired glomerular function in HIV patients treated with tenofovir. AIDS 2009;23:689–96.
58. Del Palacio M, Romero S, Casado JL. Proximal tubular renal dysfunction or damage in HIV-infected patients. AIDS Rev 2012;14:179–87.
59. Rifkin B, Perazella M. Tenofovir-associated nephrotoxicity: Fanconi syndrome and renal failure. Am J Med 2004;117:282–4.
60. Karras A, Lafaurie M, Furco A, et al. Tenofovir-related nephrotoxicity in HIV-infected patients: three cases of renal failure, Fanconi syndrome, and nephrogenic diabetes insipidus. Clin Infect Dis 2003;36:1070–3.
61. Bedimo R, Maalouf N, Zhang S, et al. Osteoporotic fracture risk associated with cumulative exposure to tenofovir and other antiretroviral agents. AIDS 2012;26: 825–31.
62. Chen L, Zhang Q, Yu DM, et al. Early changes of HBV quasispecies during lamivudine treatment and the correlation with antiviral efficacy. J Hepatol 2009;50: 895–905.
63. Chang M, Chien R, Yeh C, et al. Virus and transaminase levels determine the emergence of drug resistance during long-term lamivudine therapy in chronic hepatitis B. J Hepatol 2005;43:72–7.

64. Koklu S, Tuna Y, Gulsen M, et al. Long-term efficacy and safety of lamivudine, entecavir, and tenofovir for treatment of hepatitis B virus-related cirrhosis. Clin Gastroenterol Hepatol 2013;11:88–94.

65. Baxa D, Thekdi A, Golembieski A. Evaluation of anti-HBV drug resistant mutations among patients with acute symptomatic hepatitis B in the United States. J Hepatol 2013;58:212–6.

66. Kane M. Global programme for control of hepatitis B infection. Vaccine 1995;13: S47–9.

67. Schirmera P, Wintersb M, Holodniy M. HIV–HBV vaccine escape mutant infection with loss of HBV surface antibody and persistent HBV viremia on tenofovir/emtricitabine without antiviral resistance. J Clin Virol 2011;52:261–4.

68. Gandhi R, Wurcel A, Lee H, et al. Response to hepatitis B vaccine in HIV-1-positive subjects who test positive for isolated antibody to hepatitis B core antigen: implications for hepatitis B vaccine strategies. J Infect Dis 2005;191: 1435–41.

69. Rivas P, Herrero MD, Puente S, et al. Immunizations in HIV-infected adults. AIDS Rev 2007;9:173–87.

70. Launay O, van der Vliet D, Rosenberg AR, et al. Safety and immunogenicity of 4 intramuscular double doses and 4 intradermal low doses vs standard hepatitis B vaccine regimen in adults with HIV-1: a randomized controlled trial. JAMA 2011; 305:1432–40.

71. World Health Organisation. Hepatitis B vaccines: WHO position paper. Wkly Epidemiol Rec 2009;84:405–19.

72. Wedemeyer H, Heidrich B, Manns MP. Hepatitis D virus infection—not a vanishing disease in Europe! Hepatology 2007;45:1331–2.

73. Soriano V, Grint D, d'Arminio-Monforte A, et al. Hepatitis delta in HIV-infected individuals in Europe. AIDS 2011;25:1987–92.

74. Calle-Serrano B, Manns MP, Wedemeyer H. Hepatitis delta and HIV infection. Semin Liver Dis 2012;32:120–9.

75. Kew M. Hepatitis viruses (other than hepatitis B and C viruses) as causes of hepatocellular carcinoma: an update. J Viral Hepat 2013;20:149–57.

76. Farci P, Niro G. Clinical features of hepatitis D. Semin Liver Dis 2012;32:228–36.

77. Erhardt A, Gerlich W, Starke C, et al. Treatment of chronic hepatitis D with pegylated interferon-a 2b. Liver Int 2006;26:805–10.

78. Yurdaydin C. Treatment of chronic delta hepatitis. Semin Liver Dis 2012;32: 237–44.

79. Farci P, Roskams T, Chessa L, et al. Long-term benefit of interferon a therapy of chronic hepatitis D: regression of advanced hepatic fibrosis. Gastroenterology 2004;126:1740–9.

80. Niro G, Ciancio A, Gaeta G, et al. Pegylated interferon alpha 2b as monotherapy or in combination with ribavirin in chronic hepatitis D. Hepatology 2006;44: 713–20.

81. Yurdaydin C, Bozkaya H, Onder F, et al. Treatment of chronic d hepatitis with lamivudine vs lamivudine+ interferon vs interferon. J Viral Hepat 2008;15: 314–21.

82. Wedemeyer H, Yurdaydìn C, Dalekos G, et al, HIDIT Study Group. Peginterferon plus adefovir versus either drug alone for hepatitis delta. N Engl J Med 2011; 364:322–31.

83. Sheldon J, Ramos B, Toro C, et al. Does treatment of hepatitis B virus (HBV) infection reduce hepatitis delta virus (HDV) replication in HIV-HBV-HDV-coinfected patients? Antivir Ther 2008;13:97–102.

84. Farci P. Treatment of chronic hepatitis D: new advances, old challenges. Hepatology 2006;44:536–9.
85. Roche B, Samuel D. Liver transplantation in delta virus infection. Semin Liver Dis 2012;32:245–55.

Index

Note: Page numbers of article titles are in **boldface** type.

A

Antiviral therapy
    for chronic HBV infection
        direct antiviral therapy, 415–420
            impact on HCC development, 416–419
            impact on hepatic fibrosis, 415–416
            impact on liver disease progression, decompensation, and survival, 416
        HBsAg seroclearance as ideal outcome in, 420
        IFN-based, 414–415
    for end-stage HBV liver disease, 453–456

C

Cirrhosis
    HBV
        decompensated
            treatment of, 451–473
        in HCC, 385–389. *See also* Hepatocellular carcinoma (HCC), HBV infection in,
            treatment algorithms in, in patients with cirrhosis
            decompensated
                treatment of, **451–473**

E

Entecavir
    for chronic HBV infection
        long-term results of, 447–448

H

HBsAg. *See* Hepatitis B surface antigen (HBsAg)
HBV infection. *See* Hepatitis B virus (HBV) infection
HCC. *See* Hepatocellular carcinoma (HCC)
HDV. *See* Hepatitis D virus (HDV)
Hepatitis B surface antigen (HBsAg)
    quantification of
        in predicting natural history and treatment outcome in chronic HBV patients, **399–412**
            add on therapy, 407
            clinical applications of, 400
            described, 400–401
            HDV, 407
            natural history, 401–403

Clin Liver Dis 17 (2013) 503–506
http://dx.doi.org/10.1016/S1089-3261(13)00052-4
1089-3261/13/$ – see front matter © 2013 Elsevier Inc. All rights reserved.

liver.theclinics.com

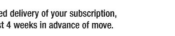